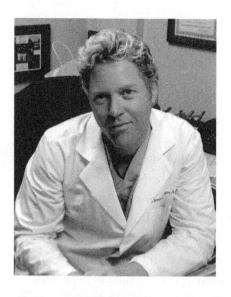

Hello! I am Dr Thomas Cangiano. Since my medical school and residency training in Urology at the University of Pennsylvania and subsequent Urologic Oncology education at the University of California at Los Angeles, I have been treating patients with a wide variety of urologic conditions in the Orlando area for over 21 years. About 10 years ago I found myself with a noticeable lack of energy, decreased libido and generally in a mental fog. It was hard to explain I just knew something was wrong. At that time very little was known about testosterone and its impact on the male. In fact, the range of testosterone considered normal was a whopping 200 to almost 900! So the scientific community was way behind the times and really unsure what was "normal" or even acceptable. All of our training as urologists and even endocrinologists was rigid and behind the times. The anti- aging community had discovered benefits of testosterone and other hormonal balances which we as urologists viewed as alternative unproven medicine since there was no real scientific proof with carefully structured studies. The problem was again that the science lagged behind the clinical conditions and many patients weren't being optimized or simply ignored when they had complaints of low libido, poor erections, reduced muscle mass, depression, moodiness, and lack of energy. Through a friend, I met an anti-aging specialist who took the time to educate me on what some of the cutting edge techniques they used to maximize hormones and make life more fulfilling. In fact, when my blood level was tested, my testosterone was considered "normal" by all standards but I knew I was not optimized. I knew I just was not feeling right. I would exercise and eat right and was getting nowhere. I tried low carbohydrate diet, you name it and just could not lose weight or gain muscle mass. I was also not necessarily in a mental fog but certainly not on my game or on point mentally. All I wanted to do was come home (sure after a stressful day) and lay on the couch and watch tv. I had lost my motivation to workout and just seemed to have lost my sharpness and creativity.

So I started a journey of being treated over 10 years ago when there was little data, little science to back all of this up. Some of it was street science. Some of it trial and error. I became my own experiment and had to learn as I went. I researched and searched for answers. The journey was long and initially it was frustrating because I could not find data to support what I felt, how I felt or how I managed myself. I would go to conferences and lectures only to find the old teachings. Our Urological Association was behind the times as was our endocrinology colleagues. So through trial and error and personal experience I was able to get ahead of the curve. I was pleased when I saw more and more studies corroborating what I knew and felt and saw first hand the advancement in the study of male aging and low T. Many of my colleagues would call me with questions but wouldn't prescribe the medication because they were afraid to. I guided them, through personal experience into uncharted waters but as the science caught up as the field evolved and our knowledge matured; we as Urologists became more aggressive in treating this condition. Billboards and radio ads began to pop up. Morning talk shows are openly discussing the topic. The most attended lectures in our annual meeting are the ones on Testosterone and the aging male. In fact, I went to one of these lectures recently and it was standing room only, probably a fire hazard for people in a closed door lecture hall.

I looked at the educational literature out there and was not satisfied. I wanted to set the record straight. I wanted to dispel the many myths I hear everyday and update you on the salient points of the current literature. I wanted something anyone and everyone could understand. Lastly, I wanted to try to simplify the nebulous and most complex male hormonal issues into simple terms.

ABOUT THE EDITOR

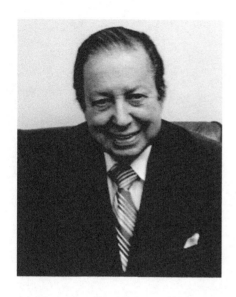

Dr Jose Cangiano has been Professor of Medicine in San Juan, Puerto Rico for over 50 years. He has focused his life work on research of hypertension and diabetes, especially in the elderly. His recent interest in hormones and the aging male complements his keen interest and expertise in bio-physiology of the aging male. He has written too many to count journal articles, publications and chapters in books. He has given hundreds of professorial lectures throughout the world in the field of aging male diseases, including hypertension, diabetes and obesity. He still practices full time and teaches in the fields of Internal Medicine and Nephrology.

the
MYTHS
— *and* —
REALITY
— *of* —
TESTOSTERONE

THOMAS CANGIANO MD

ESC PUBLISHING, LLC
St Petersburg, Florida

Disclaimer

This book is intended to educate and supplement, not replace, the advice of a well-trained physician or health professional. Every person and patient are different, so the contents of this book may not be for all men or for any individual man. The author, editor and publisher specifically disclaim any liability, loss, or risk, personal or otherwise, that is incurred as a consequence, directly or indirectly, of the use and application of any contents of the information in this book.

ESC Publishing, LLC
3614 Casablanca Ave Suite 1000
St Petersburg FL 33706

All registered trademarks in this book are the property of their respective owners

The publisher is not responsible for websites, their content or any other media social or otherwise that is not owned by the publisher

ISBN: 978-1-7334270-0-5 (HB)
ISBN: 978-1-7334270-2-9 (PB)
ISBN: 978-1-7334270-1-2 (EB)

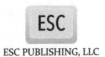

ESC PUBLISHING, LLC

Dedication

This book is dedicated to my daughter Elliana Sirena. By the time you can comprehend what is in this, it might have gone through ten editions. Hopefully, one day, the family baton of medicine will be passed to you.

Love, Papi.

SPECIAL ACKNOWLEDGMENT

I express my deepest gratitude to my fiancé, B Moree for your vision
and belief this could be done. Not only did you give me the best
gift of our daughter but you pushed me to be better and achieve my
goals- our goals. Without you this would have never been completed.
Thank you for always believing in me. We accomplished it!

ACKNOWLEDGMENTS

There are certain people in life that make an impression on you. My dad, Jose (the editor) and mother, Marilyn always taught me that with hard work and diligence you can accomplish anything. My family Joe, Lizette and Michelle who never let me take myself too seriously. My counselor and life coach Dr Eric Hennig who helped me strive to self-realize and self-actualize. Arthur Angelo for formatting and the wonderful cover and Emily Hromi for the perfect illustrations. My practice staff and colleagues who encouraged me along the way. And lastly, all of my patients who I have treated over the years who trusted me to help them live a better life.

CONTENTS

FOREWORD BY THE EDITOR

It is a most rewarding experience to participate in the elaboration of this simple and practical guide to improve your health and well-being. In my 60 years of practicing medicine, the topic of sexual performance by patients has gone from taboo to a more open, uninhibited conversation by physicians and patients regarding erectile dysfunction (ED). It is well known that this is a common condition in males. The prevalence of ED has been reported as high as 52% and increases with age. It is 40% at age 40 and as high as 70% at age 70. It is not just a condition of older males as younger males are also affected which can be a devastating phenomenon.

In my practice, I see young and elderly males with diabetes, high blood pressure, heart disease, renal failure, obesity and prostatic conditions. These are known risk factors for ED especially in younger males. As our population receives a bolus of aging males (the baby boomers) this disease will likely become more prevalent.

As our understanding of ED has evolved so has our comprehension of hypogonadism or low Testosterone and its role in male aging. We know that derangement of testosterone may be associated with a syndrome of fatigue or tiredness, lack of energy, muscular wasting, increased fat distribution, moodiness, depression, poor cognition and ED. However, there are many myths and misperceptions in the lay community about testosterone treatment and associated risks with that treatment.

In this publication, Dr Thomas Cangiano clearly presents in a simple and succinct manner the myths and reality of many testosterone misconceptions. This is especially relevant in the age of widely available and internet-based plethora of products touting to be "Testosterone boosters". His personal view and extensive experience treating patients with low testosterone stands him in good stead for making this publication. The reader may find a truthful, didactic and evidence-based prescription to alleviate this at times catastrophic milieu of symptoms associated with this condition. Notwithstanding, I hope it will serve as a trigger to a better understanding of this very common male malady.

Jose L Cangiano MD

INTRODUCTION

All of the chapters were written for hopefully, anyone to understand. They were written from someone who has personally experienced the highs and lows of testosterone, literally. Someone who has treated thousands of patients with this condition. While writing this book, the most up to date research and science was also incorporated in each of the sections. The myths were developed from so many misperceptions of Testosterone boosters and natural foods and products and even misconceptions of colleagues when treating low Testosterone. I wanted to debunk the myths, and then give real practical advice based on medicine and science. It is not a manual just for testosterone replacement and maximizing every workout and muscle fiber strength gain - I will leave that to the steroid gurus.

This is also not by any means a comprehensive manual of all the nuances of testosterone and the science behind it. Testosterone pathways and effects are very complicated even for physicians to understand so I don't really expect that anyone reading this to fully grasp how every hormone feedback loop works. There is a little science discussed here - note the short chapter on science.

Another thing to note: not all men who have low testosterone as natural process of aging need treatment. Some men with low testosterone have no symptoms or signs at all. There are debates whether this natural decline in testosterone truly causes health problems or is a an associated phenomenon with health issues like metabolic syndrome and heart disease. For those men who have the classic symptoms and signs of low energy, fatigue, decreased libido, erectile dysfunction, increased fat, reduced muscle mass and moodiness or mental fog, this book is for you!

The life expectancy of males is increasing and as such, expectations of quantity and quality of life also have increased. Expectations of a fulfilling life including sexual and mental function have become the norm. Furthermore, we are encountering a population that is the most active, health conscious and physically fit (the baby boomers) which makes this an ideal time and forum to educate as many as possible about continuing to maximize hormonal health and life satisfaction as we age.

For me, this has been a journey, and yes a very personal one. Concepts which I thought were true because of previous teachings and dogma were disproven. In doing the research for this book, I learned a good amount of facts to support the treatment I have been providing and believed in. Nonetheless, I also learned about things that I thought were true and turned out not be.

Hopefully this book will help you through your journey for better health through hormones. What you will notice is a constant theme of not just elevating your hormones to the highest possible levels but achieving *balance* with *your hormones* - like everything else in life…

So let's get you off of the bench and back into the game!

Thomas Cangiano MD FACS

the
MYTHS
— *and* —
REALITY
— *of* —
TESTOSTERONE

**A SIMPLE AND PRACTICAL GUIDE TO
GET YOU BACK IN THE GAME!**

Chapter 1

TESTOSTERONE: WHAT DOES IT DO?

Myth:

Testosterone causes cancer, makes you crazy, and if you have an enlarged prostate or heart disease, forget it...

Reality:

Testosterone has many benefits, will not make you crazy, won't cause you anymore urinary symptoms, and seems to protect the heart.

Testosterone controls:

- Libido or sex drive
- Erectile function
- Lean muscle mass
- Fat distribution
- Cognition
- Mood
- Bone mass
- Cardiac function
- Insulin sensitivity
- Fertility
- Lipid profile

MYTHS AND LEGENDS

Where do we begin? Well let's begin with dispelling all the myths. In each chapter, I will discuss and dispel the myths that are current misconceptions. In my practice I hear so many, especially the perceived reality of naturopathic remedies. I will also simplify treatment options practically because so much has changed and revolves around not just clinical effectiveness but price, practicality of life and the elephant in the room - insurance coverage. This is for the anyone who wants to understand about why low Testosterone (T) is occurring, how it can help them live a better life and how to optimally treat it.

Testosterone controls so much more than we know in the aging male. Of course, the areas of libido or sex drive, fertility and muscle and bone mass are well known. The lesser known effects especially on the male brain have yet to be truly confirmed. However, we are finding out more and more about the effects on memory, cognition, task performance, mood, including anxiety and depression, creativity and sleep patterns.

In fact, I will go over the latest studies but my experience tells me many men have subtle changes unbeknownst to them. Their partners may notice differences before they do. Some of these are minor but some become more pronounced. What I have seen over the last 10 years of treating patients is that more and more patients and doctors are becoming aware of low T and its implications in the aging male. Even the spouses and significant others know about it.

So why is it so prevalent? Is it just our awareness that has heightened or is this disease process truly becoming more prevalent. I think it is a combination. We know that after a man turns thirty his testosterone declines every year a certain percentage point. At age 30, 30% of men will have low testosterone and at age 80 it will be 70%. The over 65 male population is going to rise to 31 million in 2030 and approximately 50-60 percent of these men have low T.

We are also seeing younger and younger men who suffer the effects of low T, so what is going on? Well it is really unclear, my personal opinion and that of many health experts is that it is a combination of factors. Diet, especially high in processed foods, exercise or lack thereof, and stress play huge roles. There are chemicals and preservatives in processed and packaged foods, hormones and antibiotics in our meat supply. We also lead a sedentary lifestyle and carry tremendous daily stress in our western society which releases other hormones that fight our testosterone function and raises estrogen in males.

When our male hormones get out of balance at a young age all of those environmental factors accelerate the process of internal aging-Your organs produce less of the hormones and respond less to any and all available hormones. Also get this, many of these changes are irreversible - once they happen, it is done. Some of these changes of production and response occur slowly and are subtle so by the time you realize what is going on it becomes more difficult to deal with.

But there is hope for all men! Science has caught up with the street and patient signs and symptoms. So let's get started on our journey to hormone health and inform you about Testosterone, treatment options and dispel the myths.

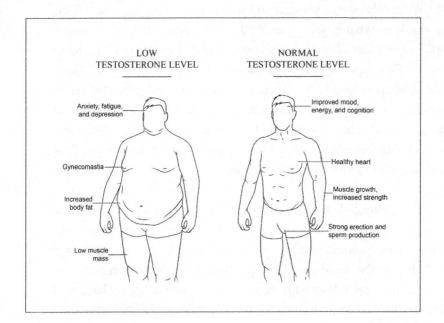

LOW
TESTOSTERONE LEVEL

NORMAL
TESTOSTERONE LEVEL

Anxiety, fatigue,
and depression

Gynecomastia

Increased
body fat

Low muscle
mass

Improved mood,
energy, and cognition

Healthy heart

Muscle growth,
increased strength

Strong erection and
sperm production

TAKE HOME POINT

*The prevalence of Low T is rising in all generations but there is hope
for all of us*

SCIENCE OF TESTOSTERONE (MADE SIMPLE)

The Magical Pathway

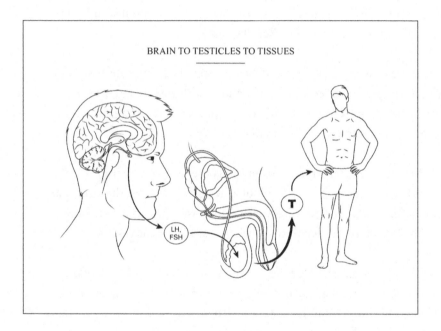

BRAIN TO TESTICLES TO TISSUES

I don't want to dwell on the science but those of you who want to know how the cascade works - its simple (well not really), but I will simplify it for you.

The hypophyseal pituitary axis (HPPS) is the magical brain pathway in which testosterone is produced. Yes this is hard to pronounce but here is what happens in simple terms. Deep in the brain a small gland called the hypophysis is responsible for producing a releasing hormone that produces many hormones but the most important is Luteinizing Hormone (LH) and the other is Follicle Stimulating Hormone (FSH). LH is responsible for testosterone production and FSH for sperm production in the male. The LH stimulates special cells in the testicle called Leydig cells to produce testosterone in the testicle. (See diagram)

As testosterone is produced it is released into the stream where it may or may not combine with protein to be bound or not, traveling to tissues. Serum hormone binging globulin (SHBG) binds testosterone and essentially disengages it from use. When it is bound it simply can't be used by the target tissues. (See diagram)

There is also a conversion of Testosterone to Dihydrotestosterone which is important in certain tissues and we will get into later. Suffice to say the free testosterone, which is only 1 or 2 percent of the circulating Testosterone, is the *gold!*, The stuff our body really uses.

Maximizing your free testosterone is the best way to improve the overall function of what we think of as testosterone. Yes, the stuff that works- that controls libido, erections, lean muscle mass, fat distribution and the typical things we think of when testosterone is discussed.

There are a bunch of feedback loops and tight control of all of these pathways, and guess what, all of these pathways can become disrupted causing low functional Testosterone. There are many times patients come in with a "normal" testosterone but the free Testosterone, their *gold*, is low. So it is important to be placed on the correct medications and obtain the correct blood work.

Interestingly, most of the young men who have issues with low testosterone are secondary to disruption of the brain axis due to unknown causes. Primary testicle issues or testicular failure may be from medications toxic to the testicles but also carry a degree of unknown causes.

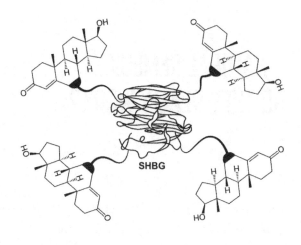

TESTOSTERONE MOLECULE BOUND TO SHBG

SHBG

TAKE HOME POINT

*The brain controls the signals to the testicles
to make Testosterone*

Chapter 3

NATURAL REMEDIES DO THEY REALLY WORK?

Myth:

Natural supplements like those T-boosters seen on TV and internet will raise my testosterone and improve my male function

Reality:

Testosterone boosters have no proven clinical effects and disingenuous reviews on websites propagate this misperception.

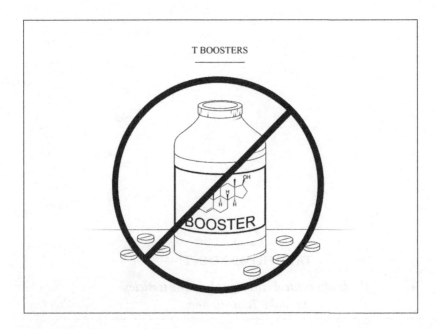

Before we go into pharmaceutical treatment options let us explore what is known or out there in our medical literature about natural remedies.

Many of you may not remember a natural herbal remedy that was introduced years ago. It was called Enzyte® and had a great marketing campaign. A man -Smilin' Bob - was smiling and waving to his wife all happy intimating he was taking the medication for "natural male enhancement". Herbal products do not require testing for ingredients or purity by the US Food and Drug Administration (FDA). The owner of the company made millions until eventually the federal government caught up with them for fabricated enhancement claims since there was no scientific evidence that substantiated their claims. That's why if you ever listen to the radio and hear an ad for a natural substance that may boost or enhance male performance the fast-talking disclaimer guy usually follows with "These statements and products have not been evaluated by the FDA, this product is not meant to diagnose, treat, cure or prevent any disease...". Testosterone boosters are no different.

Testosterone boosters have long been touted to increase muscle mass, improve energy, and burn fat. It has been shown that only just over 10 percent of T boosters have human studies to support their claims. Many of these T boosters have supra-therapeutic doses of recommended daily allowances of vitamins and minerals to compensate for the fact they have no positive effects on T.

There are so many testosterone boosters on the market it is a difficult task to separate them. Unfortunately, most supplements have little if no scientific evidence that they work. They also may come from less than reliable sources. Not only is there no proven studies to demonstrate their effectiveness, they may be harmful!

There are case reports of liver injury from ingestion of these testosterone boosters. Any of the over-the-counter supplements may be contaminated with actual anabolic steroids which when taken by mouth have a higher risk of liver injury. These boosters are at times lined with testosterone and if ingested, the liver will break them down causing damage and even liver failure. Stay away from boosters, there is no need to take them when there are legitimate real world solutions out there.

──────────── TAKE HOME POINT ────────────

Natural supplement T booster claims are disingenuous, have supra-therapeutic doses of vitamins and minerals to compensate for lack of effect on T and occasionally harmful.

Chapter 4

OTHER NATUROPATHIC SUBSTANCES: ARE THEY EFFECTIVE?

Dehydroepiandrosterone (DHEA)

Myth:

DHEA supplementation is just an oral form of testosterone and is the fountain of youth

Reality:

DHEA supplementation has not been shown to raise testosterone in men

Dehydroepiandrosterone is an androgen steroid produced by the adrenal gland or peripheral organs. The body converts it to estrogen and testosterone and other hormones and peptides. Oral DHEA supplementation has been shown to increase testosterone in women but NOT in men. Oral supplementation also increases estradiol in men and women. In men, this can be a bad thing if estradiol goes too high. Furthermore, supplemental DHEA is touted to reduce abdominal fat and may do that through other hormones or ratios of testosterone and other hormones but this is still is unclear, very controversial and unproven. It has unclear dangers when taken long term.

Side effects can include excess sweating, breast growth in men, nausea and flushing of the face. Overall, as a supplement for Testosterone elevation, DHEA has **not** been shown to elevated testosterone levels in men significantly unlike in women. Currently its anti-aging effects are as controversial as are its testosterone raising properties.

ANDROSTENEDIONE (ANDRO)

Myth:

Oral Androstenedione increases serum Testosterone concentrations

Reality:

Oral Androstenedione has not been found to increase Testosterone levels at safe manufacturer doses but larger doses beyond considered safe may increase Testosterone temporarily

The notoriety of Androstenedione peaked when several major league baseball players who were breaking long-standing home run records, admitted to using the substance. At the time it was available over-the-counter and not considered an anabolic steroid. However, due to the dangers of unregulated Testosterone and potential side effects, the Anabolic Steroid Control Act of 2004 declared androstenedione a controlled substance and banned it for over the counter purchase.

Androstenedione is a precursor of testosterone molecule. It is available in oral form and the original patent was for 50 mg to 100 mg. It was claimed to raise serum testosterone significantly up to around 100% when 100 mg were taken. Unfortunately, these claims were unfounded. It was found, however, that large doses above able the manufacturer recommended dose of 100 mg did raise testosterone transiently for 8 hours or so. The percent rise depended on the dose. If 200 mg was used on average it raised the testosterone 15% and if 300 mg used it raised the testosterone on average 30 percent. It is unclear exactly how it raises the serum Testosterone levels but it is clear that it is metabolized by the liver. Therefore, the effectiveness of the medication is raising serum testosterone depends on how far you saturate the liver and how much escapes metabolism or breakdown by the liver. Currently Andro is not available for purchase or use in the United States.

ZINC

Myth:

Zinc is only for the immune system

Reality:

Zinc is dietary mineral that is a strong natural booster of testosterone and reduces estrogen production.

Zinc has been found to boost natural testosterone and also inhibit aromatization (or conversion) of testosterone to estradiol. It has been shown that patients who have Zinc deficiency have lower testosterone.Several studies show that zinc supplementation can raise testosterone levels in testosterone deficient men with normal testosterone producing organs. 30 - 50 mg of zinc picolinate or zinc gluconate from a reliable source usually suffices to optimize testosterone production an enjoy other health benefits of Zinc.

VITAMIN D

Myth:

Vitamin D supplementation raises Testosterone levels

Reality:

Vitamin D is essential but has not been proven to raise testosterone levels

There is overwhelming evidence to suggest Vitamin D supplementation does not significantly raise serum testosterone levels. Vitamin D deficiency, however, can lead to imbalances that affect the formation of all hormones including testosterone. Further study is warranted to understand the exact relationship of this. For now, Vitamin D supplementation has not been shown to raise serum testosterone levels significantly.

EXERCISE AND TESTOSTERONE

Myth:

Aerobic exercise increases testosterone

Reality:

Resistance exercise only increases testosterone transiently

Exercise has long been thought to boost testosterone in men. It is unclear if it actually boosts testosterone or helps disassociates the free from the serum hormone binding globulin total protein. Unfortunately, this result is temporary. With weight lifting testosterone can increase but only for a short period of time.

Exercise increases DHT (one of the proteins used in target tissues) which may have greater health benefits when considering prostate cancer risk, body fat, heart disease and bone mass. Exercise lowers body fat and improves insulin sensitivity, which also may help stabilize the balance of Testosterone/Estrogen ratio. Interestingly, exercise also increases Serum Hormone Binding Globulin limiting free testosterone. So you can see just how your body keeps itself in balance.

——————————— TAKE HOME POINT ———————————

It is difficult to raise testosterone with any natural supplement or exercise consistently long term.

Chapter 5

SLEEP DISTURBANCES AND TESTOSTERONE

Myth:

Sleep is not important for hormone balance

Reality:

Sleep disturbances affects the pathways creating Testosterone imbalances and the major daily blood release of Testosterone is controlled by sleep.

Sleep is an active rather than passive process and the average sleep duration has decreased over the last several decades. In addition, the current population works longer hours with a demanding schedule, resulting in more insomnia and sleep disturbances than previous generations. Furthermore, a growing number of the population have developed obstructive sleep apnea secondary to obesity and age which affects sleep duration.

Testosterone levels are higher in the morning after sleeping. This was thought to part of the rhythmic production of hormones called the circadian rhythm. However, it has been found that this elevation is highly dependent on sleep. In fact, the major daily blood release of testosterone actually occurs during sleep. This is why blood draws for testosterone are usually recommended in the morning when the testosterone is usually highest.

It has been shown at least 3-4 hours of quality normal architecture sleep is necessary for maximal testosterone production and release. Although many of you may be thinking "well I get more sleep than that". The issue is with quality and uninterrupted sleep. Many people don't get that much uninterrupted sleep even in an eight-hour period. The average person sleeps about 6-8 hours but of that total, only a portion is considered of normal architecture or high quality. The quality and depth of the sleep is that with cycles of rapid eye movements (REM), nocturnal awakenings, and non rapid eye movement sleep. Think about how any times you tossed and turned in the evening only to realize for eight hours you truly only slept half of that because of your inability to achieve deep sleep. This deep sleep is required for that testosterone release for your day. So even if you are young, sleep disturbances and/or restriction will cause lower serum testosterone levels. It is interesting that the time of day of sleep does not matter, whether evening or daytime, as long as sleep was deep and not fragmented and of adequate length.

Obstructive Sleep Apnea (OSA) is medical condition associated with age and obesity. It is a phenomenon that occurs when the airway gets obstructed during sleep causing episodes of apnea and hypoxia (low oxygen levels). This in turn, causes a disruption in the sleep cycle. As one can imagine this condition has been associated with lower testosterone levels due to decrease secretion of Testosterone during sleep. In patients who have used a positive pressure (CPAP) machine there has been shown to be correction of their Testosterone levels to near more normal.

Here is also an interesting fact, we know sleep disturbances can affect testosterone production but also abnormal Testosterone low or high, can in turn, affect sleep quality. Men who have low Testosterone have been shown to have significant sleep disturbances including insomnia independent of age. Also men with too high of testosterone levels have been shown to suffer from insomnia as well. Each one is interdependent and can affect the other.

So high quality sleep of adequate duration is required for any individual to restore energy and Testosterone.

Sleep conditions that affect quality sleep and subsequent Low T

- **Insomnia**
- **Sleep apnea**
- **Stress**

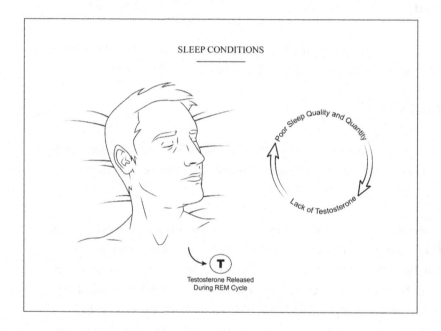

SLEEP CONDITIONS

Poor Sleep Quality and Quantity

Lack of Testosterone

Testosterone Released
During REM Cycle

—————————— TAKE HOME POINT ——————————

Quality sleep is the most important factor for adequate daily testosterone release.

Chapter 6

LEGITIMIZE YOUR THERAPY - GET OFF THE GYM JUICE!

Myth:

The only way you can really get in shape is by buying illegal steroids on the internet or the gym manufactured in China

Reality:

There are plenty of safe and viable pharmaceutical grade options with quality control that can be used to restore or replace testosterone safely

Let's talk about the street science - and this time be honest. So this chapter is for those of you who have been seeking more but going at it the wrong way. This is for all of you at the gym following the blogs, friends, family, Dr Google and street science. For those of you perhaps obtaining your medications from unclear and maybe dubious sources. From the internet, China, Mexico and any health professional not certified in medicine as we know it.

Anabolic steroids and steroid abuse is more commonplace now than ever before. It was once reserved for only the athletes seeking increased endurance and strength. Subtle modifications to the testosterone molecule can make them more powerful and effective but also more dangerous. Our bodies were not meant to have supra-physiological levels of testosterone and as such, significant side effects and complications can arise. Many of these consequences are irreversible. Trenbolone, Sustanon, Nalondrone just to name a few, are the highly anabolic steroids with significant side effects and at times dangerous long term permanent effects. (see below)

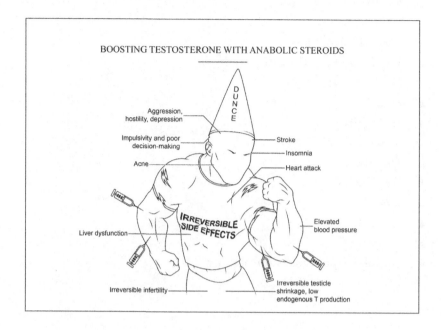

I have patients who come in on illegitimate medication, unsafe medication and are tired of the clandestine process. They want to be legitimized. I tell them I am willing to do it but on my terms. No more street science. Yes I am clearly in tune to all of the street blogs and titration of mixtures of multiple agents to seemingly maximize their results. I tell them I am a licensed physician, and as such I need to follow the rules of what we know. Yes, I can use medications off label but it needs to be clear that we will not exceed the boundaries of what is deemed safe. In fact, keeping you safe and healthy while maximizing your hormone results is my goal.

So those of you doing a little of this and that and on your own concoctions bought at the gym forcing labs, be true to yourself and your families. Consult with your physician and perhaps an expert in the field of urology or endocrinology to help you through your journey of good, safe health and hormonal balance.

Risks with Gym juice :

- Liver dysfunction
- Elevated Blood Pressure
- Heart Attack
- Stroke
- Infertility
- Mood changes
- Depression
- Aggression
- Hostility
- Acne
- Insomnia
- Impulsive poor decision-making

TAKE HOME POINT

Anabolic steroids are dangerous and may cause irreversible side effects

RESTORING VS REPLACEMENT - WHICH IS THE BEST OPTION?

Myth:

Testosterone needs to be always be replaced if low

Reality:

Many times if the testicles are still working we can boost them with medication restoring the testicle function

B oosting your own natural testosterone is one of the most common and natural ways to raise your testosterone and restore it. So the first question I ask men is if they want more children. Why is this important? Because back in the day we didn't understand the true effects on fertility. Testosterone replacement therapy (as opposed to restorative therapy) was being used and patients were not being told or were unaware that replacing T would actually reduce their own natural T leading to lower sperm costs and infertility. The complex need for a pulsatile rather than continuous elevated Tis necessary for optimal sperm production. So many of these men treated were sub fertile or even infertile and at times it was irreversible.

I have found over the years that if I can still boost a man's own natural testosterone and adequately adjust his levels, I see less side effects of estrogen imbalance and elevated dangerous blood counts. Also fertility remains intact which is really important for men with low testosterone who want to remain fertile. So in that vain there are two fertility medications that are currently used off label but gaining more widespread usage in daily practice for low T. One is clomiphene citrate (Clomid) and the other is human chorionic gonadotropin (HCG).

—————————————— TAKE HOME POINT ——————————————

Before just replacing your T, ask your doctor about trying to stimulate the testicles to restore your T level

Chapter 8

CLOMIPHENE CITRATE

Myth:

Clomiphene is only used for female infertility to increase egg production

Reality:

Clomiphene is used off label to stimulate testosterone production

Clomiphene citrate (Clomid) was widely used a a fertility medication to increase ovulation (egg production) in the female. It is a selective estrogen receptor modulator and through a feedback loop raises the brain hormones - Follicle Stimulating Hormone (FSH) and Luteinizing Hormone (LH). These in turn stimulate the testicles to make testosterone and more sperm production. Clomiphene requires functioning testicles since it makes the testicles make more of its own natural testosterone. (See diagram)

It is in pill form and the usual dosage is 50 mg every other day. I found in my practice that if a man does not respond to this within 4-6 weeks he will unlikely respond for a longer trial interval and I don't want to waste his time while he is frustrated. Furthermore, increasing the dose to daily does not seem to have a significant clinical effect in the majority of men that I have treated.

When it does work, clomiphene raises testosterone and it is a convenient pill that is relatively cheap. The problem with this therapy as single therapy is that at times it may raise estrogen significantly causing side effects and even gynecomastia or 'man boobs'. So most patients I will also treat with an estrogen blocker (aromatase inhibitor like anastrozole) because of the real significance of rising estrogen levels.

I will check blood work within 4- 6 weeks and if in range and the patient is doing well clinically then I will do a check at 4 months and every 6 months thereafter. My experience with clomiphene citrate is the many young male patients do well with this. They have an increased libido, decreased fatigue, better erections and more energy and mental clarity. In older individuals I find that even if their testosterone rises to significant levels and I mean total testosterone in the 900 ng/dL to 1100 ng/dL range, they may not feel the clinical effects. Some say they don't feel the energy or libido. It has been shown that men treated with clomiphene therapy may have decreased libido and sexual satisfaction scores. For this reason if the patient does not feel the benefit I will quickly switch them to an alternative like Human Chorionic Gonadotropin (HCG) if they want to maintain their fertility or testosterone replacement therapy if they do not.

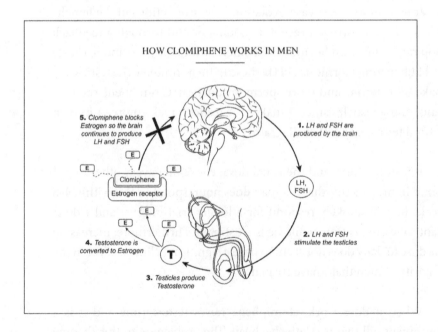

HOW CLOMIPHENE WORKS IN MEN

5. Clomiphene blocks Estrogen so the brain continues to produce LH and FSH

1. LH and FSH are produced by the brain

LH, FSH

Clomiphene

Estrogen receptor

2. LH and FSH stimulate the testicles

4. Testosterone is converted to Estrogen

3. Testicles produce Testosterone

One last note about clomiphene, it is often used by anabolic steroid users to improve their own natural production after an injectable testosterone cycle which suppresses testicle production and size so many men will try to use it off label to improve testicle recovery after a "cycle" of suppression with exogenous injectable testosterone. Although this is street science we have no data supporting safety of this but as we learn more, the safety of this strategy will become more clear.

Advantages of Clomiphene Citrate

- Oral medication
- Usually inexpensive
- Every other day dosing
- Easily portable

Disadvantages of Clomiphene Citrate

- Not very dose adjustable
- Needs intact testicle function
- High conversion of testosterone to estrogen
- High T blood levels without that feeling
- Less improvement in libido and sexual function

TAKE HOME POINT

Clomiphene is used off label to stimulate the testicles to make T with mixed results of desired effects including libido and sexual satisfaction

Chapter 9

HUMAN CHORIONIC GONADOTROPIN (HCG)

Myth:

Human Chorionic Gonadotropin (HCG) is scary and hard to deal with and just used in weight loss clinics

Reality:

HCG is very easy to use and one of the best options for patients with intact testicle function who want to raise their testosterone and maintain fertility.

Another medication that stimulates testosterone production is human chorionic gonadotropin. This is basically a medication that works like the LH and FSH to stimulate the testicles to produce testosterone and sperm.

It comes in several forms brand name and generic and recently has been very difficult to obtain because of national shortages of production. It comes in 2 vials, a lyophilized powder in one vial and sterile water to dilute it in the other vial. A solution is made with the desired concentration and injected with a small needle subcutaneously (under the skin) typically daily or every other day. This is the also medication used short term in many weight loss clinics.

I usually have patients mix 10,000 units in 10 ml of sterile water to create a concentration of 1000 units per ml. Then I will have a patient begin injecting 500 units (0.5 ml) every other day subcutaneously with a 1 cc tuberculin syringe with a 29 or 30 gauge needle. These small needles are almost painless even for patients who are wary of injections.

What is really nice about this medication is that it can be titrated, that is, dose adjusted. So if the initial dose does not work it can be raised to see if subsequent higher doses stimulate the testicles to make more testosterone. Usual increments of increase are 100 to 200 units every other day. Once again blood levels should be checked with any changes and usually within 4-6 weeks of initiating the injections. The only issue with this medication is that it needs an intact testosterone production mechanism in the testicle, is expensive, at times unavailable and not necessarily convenient for travel since it needs to be refrigerated. HCG is widely used as single therapy and has been shown to have less aromatization or conversion to estrogen, requiring less use of estrogen blockers. This has been my experience as well.

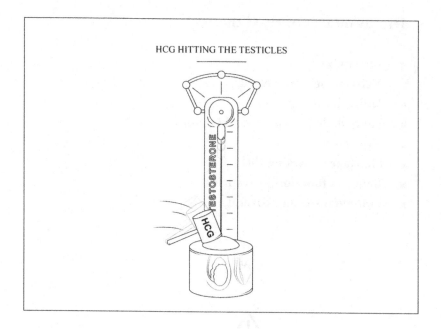

HCG HITTING THE TESTICLES

Advantages of HCG therapy

- Dose adjustable
- Effective when intact testicle function
- Injections have minimal pain- Small insulin type needs used
- Maintains fertility
- No testicle shrinkage
- Can be used in combination with testosterone injections to limit testicle atrophy
- Less prostate growth issues
- Less increase in estrogen aromatization and gynecomastia
- Less incidence of high hematocrit (high red cell count)
- May improve lipid profile

Disadvantages of HCG therapy

- Injection
- Needs to be refrigerated
- Difficult for travel
- Short shelf life once mixed (1 month)
- Expensive
- Shortages in availability
- Requires functioning testicles
- Limited insurance coverage

TAKE HOME POINT

Human Chorionic Gonadotropin is an excellent option to restore more natural T levels and is dose adjustable

Chapter 10

ESTROGEN BLOCKERS (AROMATASE INHIBITORS)

Myth:

These are anti-cancer drugs and should not be used to elevate testosterone or lower estrogen levels

Reality:

This medication is used quite frequently off-label to stimulate testosterone levels and reduce estrogen

At some point the testicles in the male begin to shut down. Trying to stimulate them by any means just won't work or function anymore. Sometimes in young men it is unclear why this happens. In younger men the pathways in the brain are commonly affected for unknown reasons and the testicles are still intact. In older men it is clear, it is a natural aging process of testicle shutting down. I have seen many young patients whose testicles have just shutdown for unknown reasons. Some of the major theories is that environmental factors caused this but again it is difficult to prove.

Both letrozole and anastrozole are estrogen receptor blockers or aromatase inhibitors. These are medications used in receptor positive breast cancer. They have been used off label to stimulate testicles through a negative feedback loop to produce more testosterone. I have seen very few patients on this single therapy strategy. Most of the patients I have treated, achieve the desired blood levels but their libido and energy do not exactly increase to desired levels. So this strategy as a single agent in my experience, has its limitations. (see below)

Advantages of Aromatase inhibitors

- Oral Medication - no needles
- Portable for travel
- Inexpensive
- No injection required
- Raises testosterone and blocks estrogen simultaneously
- No testicle shrinkage

Disadvantages of Aromatase inhibitors

- Requires intact testicles
- No dose adjustment
- High T blood levels without that feeling
- Hot flashes
- Night sweats
- Less improvement in libido and sexual function
- If go too low decrease bone mineral density

_____ TAKE HOME POINT _____

Estrogen blockers are widely used off label to raise testosterone but more so to control the potentially serious effects of high estrogen levels from aromatization of Testosterone

REPLACEMENT THERAPY

Myth:

If I replace my testosterone, I only need to be on it for a few months until my testicles take over

Reality:

Replacement therapy is likely lifelong, or as long as you want to feel the way you do on it

GELS

Myth:

Gels can be applied safely without consequence

Reality:

Extreme care must be taken now to have a gel get in the wrong hands or expose females or children

When I first started treating patients with low testosterone around 10 years ago, the most popular treatments were not testosterone boosters but patches, gels and shots. The patches were the first generation gel offered usually applied to the scrotum (yes scrotum) then to the arm. Unfortunately the patches did not have enough surface area to generate larger concentrations for adequate clinical testosterone levels and were quite irritating.

Other topical gels with newer delivery pharmacokinetics (bases for absorption) were then introduced. These were very popular for many years until the number of patients being treated became too great and insurance coverage began to dwindle rapidly. The brand names are very expensive but have patented delivery absorption bases that allow for better penetrations and increased blood levels in men. Currently many compounding pharmacies can make generic testosterone creams using a "man base" cream (as opposed to a generic or "female base" cream which have different absorption properties) which helps absorb the testosterone powder in the man's skin. They can be quite effective if the pharmacy is a reliable source of compounds.

Gels would be applied after showering to clean skin. The patient would towel off and dry then apply the gel, let it dry some and then place their shirt or in the case of thigh gels, their pants. (See diagram)

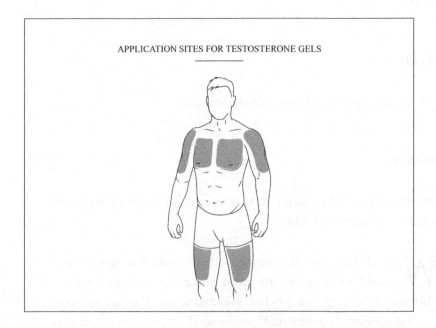

APPLICATION SITES FOR TESTOSTERONE GELS

All the gels worked usually very well and the majority of patients had significant improvement in clinical symptoms and objective blood levels if given high enough dosages of gel. Some, however, would not have clinically significant blood levels even when higher doses or more gel was applied. The skin would just not absorb the medication no matter how much was lathered on. In other patients, a small amount of cream or gel would skyrocket their testosterone levels. There was wide variance with each individual based on skin absorption and sweat with significant trial and error.

Gels are still popular today because they provide testosterone replacement daily which minimizes the peaks and valleys associated with injections. These were the most popular forms of treatment until insurances began to decline coverage and patients were being required to pay out of pocket which usually meant about six hundred dollars or so a month. As you can imagine very few could afford this. Currently many compounded gels and creams are available through compounding pharmacies. I have seen some work and some not. So if that is the route you choose, it just needs to be tried and see how the subjective symptoms and objective labs improve adjusting the dose to dial in the desired effects.

Usually, I check testosterone blood levels in 3-4 weeks after the commencement of gel application. This is usually plenty of time to see if we are getting the desired effects of the gel. Then we can adjust the dose or amount of gel to obtain the desired T blood levels and also carefully monitoring other unwanted blood levels like estrogen and too much red blood cells. One point of caution with gels is that women or children should not come in contact with the gel and they need to be placed in a safe and secure area where a young child cannot obtain access inadvertently.

Advantages of gels

- More steady levels of testosterone (less peaks and valleys)
- Easy daily application
- No shot (many men can't handle needles)
- Less conversion to estrogen

Disadvantage of gels

- Can be messy
- Daily application is time consuming
- Sweating decreases effectiveness
- Transference (Extreme caution with children and women contact to applied areas)
- May reduce fertility
- Expensive without insurance coverage
- Testicular atrophy (shrinkage)

—————————— TAKE HOME POINT ——————————

Gels and patches were popular years ago but due to current medical economics have lacked luster

TESTOSTERONE INJECTIONS

Myth:

Testosterone injections are difficult to administer and confusing

Reality:

Testosterone injections are easy, can be relatively painless if done correctly

The testosterone injection has become one of the mainstays of replacement therapy. The major reasons are that it is cheap and effective. It comes in several forms and the most widely used are testosterone cypionate and testosterone enanthate. Both come in vials of medication dissolved in oil for slower release. Historically, these injections were given monthly. A patient would come in to the doctor's office and get a shot once a month. What we found was that men felt great usually the first week but then as the medication concentration dwindled, they crashed to sub therapeutic levels for two or more weeks until the next injection. This is peculiar because the half-lives of these medications are 4-8 days. So it interesting that the initial dosing regimen was monthly which clearly was not enough.

Well then why not just give a higher dose so it lasts the whole month? The problem with that reasoning is that the initial dose would be too high sending patients into superhuman or supra-physiologic levels of testosterone with subsequent side effects and significant aromatization or conversion to estrogen. Also, their red blood cell counts would go up significantly creating more potential risk of clotting.

Typical doses of testosterone cypionate or enanthate shots are 1 cc of 200 mg/ml every 1 to 2 weeks. Smaller doses, two times per week also work well. Blood levels of free/total testosterone, estradiol and red blood cell counts are checked to ensure desired levels. These can be titrated to the desired levels and effects. It is important to obtain blood levels at the halfway point of any two injections to check for desired objective levels. The preferred delivery of the shots is intramuscular although more evidence suggests subcutaneous injections are equally safe, effective and less painful. (see below)

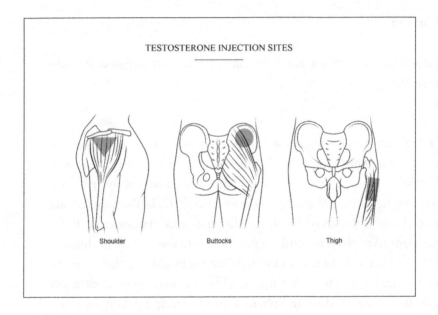

One of the last signs a patient may experience is testicular atrophy or shrinkage. The bottom line is that if you replace testosterone the testicles that were making it shrink down because of lack of use - yes if you don't use them you lose them. Some men this is bothersome and others don't really care. The reality is that I have never experienced a partner who really cares how her or his significant other's testicles appear but some men this appearance is a deal breaker. These men can inject HCG in low doses every other day to keep them plump (see chapter on testicle shrinkage).

Advantages of Testosterone shots

- Inexpensive and generic
- Widely available
- Shot every 1 or 2 weeks (not daily)
- Dose adjustable
- Intramuscular use but can also be given subcutaneously

Disadvantages of Testosterone shots

- Injection with large bore needle
- Can be painful
- Viscous solution at times difficult to withdraw
- Peaks and valleys
- High level of conversion to estrogen (aromatization)
- Travel with meds may be cumbersome
- Testicular atrophy (shrinkage)

TAKE HOME POINT

Testosterone oil injections have become popular due to ease of use, cost and availability.

TESTOSTERONE PELLETS

Myth:

Testosterone pellets are rarely used in practice

Reality:

Testosterone pellets are a great way to elevate testosterone levels with minimal side effects but may be cost prohibitive if you lack the insurance coverage

I really like the pellets as long term replacement therapy. There is a gentle rise of testosterone levels, sustainment and a subsequent slow decline over about 3 to 4 months depending on the number of pellets. A usual starting dose is 10-12 pellets placed subcutaneously in the buttock (see diagram). There is also significant advantages with stable serum levels in terms of conversion or aromatization to estrogen. Many of these men don't have significant rises in estrogen levels. The pellets are easily placed in the subcutaneously in the buttocks with a small incision with local anesthesia. Multiple pellets are inserted and blood levels checked at one month and three months until the desired levels are achieved. So why aren't these more popular and more widely used? Simple healthcare economics - too expensive and insurance coverage is now limited. There are cheaper generic alternatives for men with low testosterone regardless of foreseen benefits. If you have good insurance coverage or you can afford the pellets they are an extremely convenient and effective method to replace T limiting unwanted side effects significantly. The only issue is that you are beholden to your doctor's office to place them.

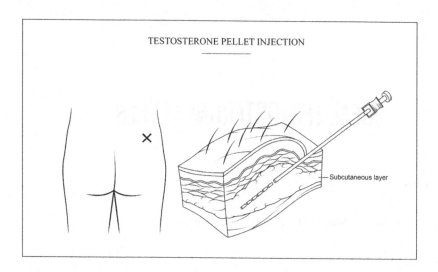

TESTOSTERONE PELLET INJECTION

Subcutaneous layer

Advantages of Pellets

- Convenient - no need to carry supplies
- Sustained testosterone levels for months
- No to little peaks or valleys
- Decreased conversion to estrogen
- Decreased incidence of high red blood cell count

Disadvantages of Pellets

- Expensive
- Limited insurance coverage
- Incision required in office
- Can overshoot without being able to "take it back"

―――――――――― TAKE HOME POINT ――――――――――

Testosterone pellets are almost an ideal way to deliver testosterone but have significant cost issues.

IDEAL TESTOSTERONE LEVELS

Myth:

The same ideal testosterone range is for all men

Reality:

There is a range of testosterone levels and each man is different, the ideal testosterone range is individual

So I am always asked after I tell a patient that they have low testosterone and the same question comes up "What should my levels be?" Or "What are my ideal levels for my age?" The answer is that there are no ideal levels or recommended levels. We know what low testosterone levels are, we know what high testosterone levels are but in the middle is a wide range we are less clear of "ideal" levels.

This is a lab value just like any other that we just don't treat to elevate without discussing signs, symptoms, and treatment outcomes. The bottom line is that each patient is different and there is no blood level that fits all men. Some men feel great at a total testosterone of 200 ng/dL. Some still feel weak with T levels in the 1000's ng/dL. The *free* testosterone is also one of most important levels to follow but is difficult to assess ideal levels for various reasons. Each lab may use a different scale - some labs use picograms per milliliter (pg/mL) and others use nanogram per deciliter (ng/dL) so it is hard for even doctors to figure out and takes some experience.

Currently most guidelines including the Urological and Endocrine community define low testosterone by total in ng/dL. Somewhere less than 300 ng/dL is considered low and other recommendations are less than 400 ng/dL. What I have found is that men with less than 400 ng/dL and signs and symptoms of low testosterone should undergo a trial of stimulation therapy or replacement therapy. Men with a normal serum testosterone level and low free testosterone level and signs and symptoms should also undergo a trial of restoration or replacement therapy. Men with low testosterone and no clinical symptoms should not routinely be offered therapy. Don't forget testosterone reduction is a natural part of aging, so the reality is that it does not need to be treated.

My Observations:

In terms of total testosterone I like most men to be between 500 and 900 ng/dL. Below 500 I find men don't really feel any difference. Above this level men feel more energetic with a desire to exercise and do activities, increased libido and come out of that mental fog. I usually start at lower doses then escalate based on experience, mode of use (gel vs pill vs injection). I will check labs frequently in the beginning every 4 weeks or so until I can dial a man in. I don't like starting men on testosterone then checking labs in 3 months. I found that with 4-6 weeks of any therapy you are going to know subjectively (by patient symptoms) and objectively (labs) whether we are going in the right direction, and the current therapy is working. If I start a man on clomiphene therapy and with in 4 -6 weeks we don't see any bump in testosterone levels, it is highly unlikely for it suddenly go up after 3 months. If I start a man on testosterone injections every 2 weeks and he is not responding or has not had a response a few days after the injection and quickly tapers down usually after a week, I will either increase the frequency of injections to weekly or bump up the dose. I prefer to increase the frequency of injections at a lower dose due to less peak and valleys and less aromatization or conversion to estrogen but some men simply cannot inject themselves that frequently.

What I don't want to happen is a man wait for 3 or 4 months for something to happen and then we get no clinical results and he feels frustrated and demoralized. I see many second opinion patients who

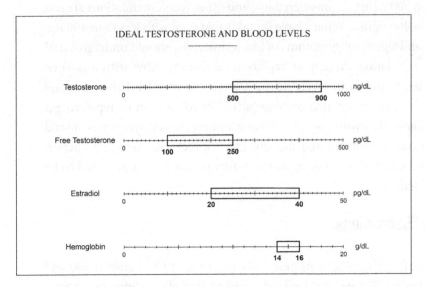

IDEAL TESTOSTERONE AND BLOOD LEVELS

have been on T therapy but just not high enough and their primary care doctor who started them on testosterone therapy does not feel comfortable increasing their dosage.

So what happens when the levels are too high. This is the part where the street and legitimate medicine diverge. Most body builders and athletes on testosterone will be at supra-physiologic levels, that is, too high usually a total testosterone level over 1100 ng/dL or a free over 250 pg/dL. Too high of levels will cause many of the symptoms and signs seen in the list of supra-physiologic effects. This is why it is important to check labs frequently in the beginning but then taper the lab schedule once stable desired levels are achieved.

It has been shown that too high of a testosterone level can cause certain side effects as listed below. Many of the physical side effects are well known as are some of the psychological side effects like aggression and hostility (aka, "Roid Rage"). Other side effects like poor cognitive reflection (not global function) or impulsivity are currently being studied and elucidated. When there is a lack of reflection on decisions and impulsivity this can lead to at times poor decision-making with high testosterone levels. Supra-physiologic T levels also decrease the threshold for risk aversion and raise the threshold for fear, conflict and stress thereby provoking more spontaneous, impulsive and utilitarian decisions which may lack moral judgement and thought-out consequences. We can see how this may affect someone close to that person *vis a vis* an interpersonal relationship but also one can extrapolate this to behaviors causing social and financial consequences of recklessness, risk- taking behavior and lack of emotion with utilitarian decisions based on outcome. There needs to be more study in this area but there is a preponderance of evidence that suggests a high or supra-physiologic T level may cause someone to make poor, impulsive decisions without well thought out consequences, among other things. (See below)

Effects of a supra-physiologic (too high) testosterone levels

- Anxiety
- Steroid psychosis or Roid Rage
- Acne
- Facial redness
- Increased Estrogen levels from aromatization leading to gynecomastia
- Possible heart attack and stroke
- Sexual Aggressiveness
- Erythrocytosis or high red blood cell count
- Sleep disturbances
- Fluid retention
- Elevated lipid profile
- Poor decision-making

TAKE HOME POINT

Ideal testosterone levels are different for every man, thats why it is important to discuss signs and symptoms and not just dwell on numbers

ERYTHROCYTOSIS: HIGH RED BLOOD CELL COUNT

Myth:

We don't need to check total blood count in men taking testosterone therapy

Reality:

It is extremely important to check red blood cell counts in men taking testosterone therapy

Unfortunately one of the side effects or peripheral effects of testosterone therapy in certain forms, especially gel and injections is erythrocytosis. This is a fancy term for high red blood cell count which will be reflected in a complete blood count (CBC). A high hemoglobin(Hb) or hematocrit is the actual lab value which becomes elevated in this blood panel. So if you are anemic or slightly anemic, testosterone therapy can help bring your red blood cell count up. Sometimes in normal men receiving testosterone the blood count goes too high. High is usually over 17 grams per deciliter (g/dL) depending on the lab. If the blood count climbs over this then it is wise to do several things. One take a baby aspirin daily to thin the blood (this is controversial since the main clotting mechanism may not be inhibited but it can perhaps hinder increased clot on top of clot). Two, if the hemoglobin goes over 17g/dL, I usually recommend blood donation or therapeutic blood draws at least once a month along with a daily aspirin. Why you may ask. If the blood count goes too high the blood becomes thicker and at times excessively thick and may increase risk of clotting.

Also, elevated red blood cells can potentially cause elevation of blood pressure which is another concern for heart attack and stroke.

So, in a patient with erythrocytosis they should also donate blood at least once a month depending on levels to get their Hb to 16 g/dL or as close to that as possible. Blood donation or therapeutic blood draws can be scheduled with the local blood donation centers. Criteria and levels for therapeutic blood draws can be scheduled in the order sheet to specify the blood levels desired.

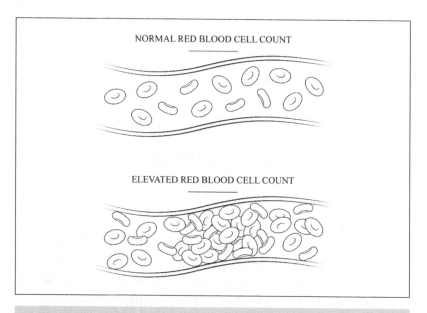

NORMAL RED BLOOD CELL COUNT

ELEVATED RED BLOOD CELL COUNT

How to deal with elevated red blood cell count

- Take a daily aspirin
- Therapeutic blood draws

TAKE HOME POINT

High red cell count can be dangerous and needs to be monitored and treated with therapeutic blood draws (blood letting)

HIGH ESTROGEN - DO YOU CRY AT MOVIES?

Myth:

Estrogens in males doesn't matter

Reality:

Optimal estrogen levels in males is crucial for libido, lowering heart risks and bone mass

Ok the title is a cheap shot but gets the point across. As I began treating males with testosterone, I was noticing estrogen levels rising. The standing joke if you have high estrogen, "Do you cry at movies?" Well I shed my tears at movies and my estrogen is exactly is where it is supposed to be. We know that if testosterone goes too high in certain males especially those with significant intra-abdominal fat, it will be converted to estrogen. You see your body does not want all this high testosterone running around, because sometimes too high makes you make bad decisions, and be too aggressive. We have all heard of "Roid Rage" or testosterone psychosis and this is a mechanism of your body to reduce too much of a good thing. There are studies that have shown that if testosterone levels are too high we as males can make bad decisions. Life decisions, financial decisions, relationship decisions - you name it. So yes, we want balance and if we live in balance, especially when considering estrogen then we can achieve many of the benefits of testosterone without the many side effects high estrogen brings. That, along with higher than normal levels of blood count making your blood thicker may play a significant role in one of the potential risks of clotting.

The side effects of high estrogen levels include, facial redness, potential inhibition of the testosterone receptor, water weight gain and clotting, Yes clotting. It has been well known that estrogen taken orally in females may increase clotting including deep vein thrombosis and subsequent pulmonary embolus which can be fatal. The same can occur in men so it is important to monitor these levels closely.

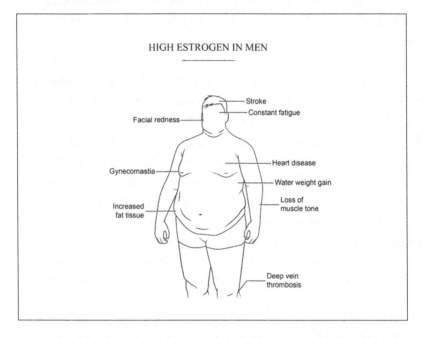

HIGH ESTROGEN IN MEN

One of the most controversial issues with testosterone replacement therapy was the increased risks of heart attack and stroke seen in a population of Veteran Administration men who took injectable testosterone replacement.This prompted the FDA in 2015 to have manufacturers of testosterone replacement therapies add a statement of increased risks of heart attack and stroke to the labels. The results of this study have since been debunked and contradicted but one could extrapolate giving a man testosterone without checking their estrogen levels may increase risk of clotting and subsequent heart attack and stroke. So there are medications to reduce the conversion of testosterone to estrogen when more conservative measures like decreasing alcohol consumption and supplemental zinc 50 mg don't work.

We don't want to just give medications to lower estrogen without identifying a goal of a level because too low of and estrogen level will reduce libido significantly and also may have long term effects on bone support growth and mass. Males need some estrogen just not too much. Really what I am trying to say again is balance. Yes the dials and levers needs to be adjusted and monitored so when testosterone goes up estrogen levels do not rise too much or fall too low when a high estrogen blood level is treated. Ideal estrogen (measured as estradiol) levels are between 20 and 40 pg/dL.

Estrogens, specifically estradiol, can increase the risk of prostate cancer in animal studies. Estradiol or too much of it has been thought to be carcinogenic. This is purported to be through a mechanism of increase inflammation on cells inducing DNA changes or direct gene changes by its metabolites and/or hormonal receptor changes causing DNA changes. We know that testosterone itself does not cause prostate cancer but certainly can make it progress once it is there. Estrogen is needed to induce and develop prostate cancer so this is another important reason to keep estradiol at normal levels. The role of anti-estrogens or aromatase inhibitors in preventing these estrogen associated changes has not been explored yet but intuitively one can see this may help.

Side effects of high Estrogen

- Facial redness,
- Inhibition of function of testosterone at the receptor level
- Water weight gain
- Potential clotting
- Potential increase risk of prostate cancer

Side effects of low Estrogen

- Decreased bone mineral repair
- Decreased libido

Things to stay away from which may create high estrogen:

- Stress
- High alcohol consumption
- Medications that raise estrogen levels
- Highly processed foods
- Bottled water or packaged foods with BPA or BPS or phthalates

─────────── TAKE HOME POINT ───────────

High estrogen can be dangerous and cause many side effects, too low estrogen will also have negative effects, especially with libido

GYNECOMASTIA - AKA "MAN BOOBS"

Myth:

Gynecomastia or "man boobs" go away with testosterone replacement

Reality:

Gynecomastia or "man boobs" are a result of estrogen to testosterone ratio imbalance and may not respond to medical therapy

This would be a good time to talk about gynecomastia or man boobs. This is usually a side effect of elevated estrogen levels that allows male breast tissue to grow. This is in distinction with breast tenderness which also is caused by imbalances in the testosterone and estrogen ratios. Obesity also makes all of this worse because of the

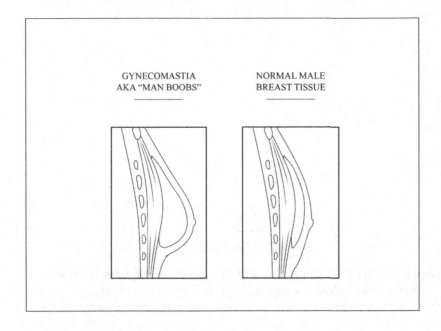

GYNECOMASTIA
AKA "MAN BOOBS"

NORMAL MALE
BREAST TISSUE

increased levels of the aromatase in fat that elevates estrogens further. The imbalance of hormones makes the breast tissue glands grow. Many times this is easily perceptible with a trained clinical eye, even in men with clothes on.

The issue with gynecomastia is that it is essentially irreversible. Once the tissue grows it usually remains and difficult to get rid of. Medical therapy is only successful in early stages of the breast tissue formation and to prevent further growth. Surgical therapy is usually required in patients looking for cosmetic improvement, so it is extremely important to keep estrogen levels normal and monitored during therapy.

—————————————— TAKE HOME POINT ——————————————

Any man on T therapy must be examined for signs of breast enlargement

TESTICLE ATROPHY (SHRINKAGE)

Myth:

Testicle atrophy affects a male negatively

Reality:

There is no negative effect of testicle atrophy other than appearance

Unfortunately as the old adage goes if you don't use it you lose it. The same thing happens with testicles. So if you take any form of replacement therapy there is a risk of testicular shrinkage or atrophy. In some men this does not bother them at all. Nonetheless, in others it seems to really affect their self-appearance and perhaps manhood. In these men, I have used a small dose of human chorionic gonadotropin once or twice weekly to maintain testicle size due to atrophy of the testosterone producing glands in the testicle. Dosages of 250 to 500 units of HCG two times weekly works well to maintain testicular volume.

—————————   **TAKE HOME POINT**   —————————

Testicle shrinkage is a cosmetic issue and causes no harm

TESTOSTERONE AND ERECTILE FUNCTION - YOU NEED GAS IN THE TANK...

Myth:

Testosterone will give you erections

Reality:

Testosterone is the gas but requires other functioning parts

We know testosterone controls sexual interest or libido. However, it was thought for some time it did not participate in erectile function, that is getting more blood flow to the penis. We know through newer studies it does more than that. Testosterone improves several things in the male penis - blood flow, smooth muscle fibers, nerve fibers and the tunica albuginea (chamber wall), tissue structure, and this last one is really important.

Let's start with blood flow. There is a misconception the penis is a muscle. It is not, it does have smooth muscle but the penis has two chambers that fill with blood to drive and maintain an erection. So, if more blood flows in than out you get and maintain an erection. If you don't have blood flowing in or you have blood flow in and it is escaping then you will not maintain an erection. Testosterone helps in all of the above.

It seems that blood flow is regulated by nerves, arteries and smooth muscle. These are some complicated processes that occur but lest to say testosterone helps nerve response thereby enhancing nitric oxide. Nitric Oxide is a powerful smooth muscle relaxer that happens to be in many tissues but also important in the penis for dilation of the arteries resulting in increased blood flow. Testosterone also seems to improve the lining of the penile arterial network allowing for better function and more dilation. **Increased Blood Flow = Better Erection**.

Back to the nitric oxide, this is also what is important in the function of the PDE 5 inhibitors also known as the little blue pill, sildenafil, and its associates. Sildenafil which was Viagra® is now generic. This medication and others work by causing relaxation of the smooth muscle arteries through increased nitric oxide in the penis to bring more blood flow in. It has been shown that Testosterone helps this performance through enhancement of its function. Hence the gas tank in the car reference. So in patients with low testosterone these oral medications may not work to their full capacity. Replacing testosterone has shown to improve PDE5 inhibitor function of increasing blood flow to the penis.

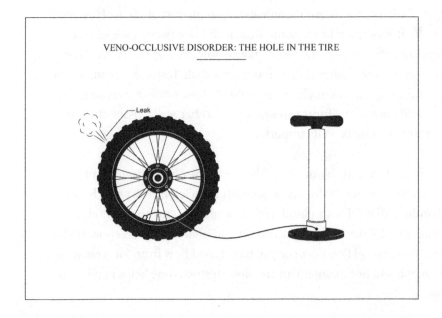

VENO-OCCLUSIVE DISORDER: THE HOLE IN THE TIRE

Leak

Lastly, have you ever tried to inflate a tire with a hole in it. You keep pumping air into the tire and it just keeps leaking out. The tunica albuginea is a layer that acts like the tire. It maintains blood flow in the penis. So many men will complain that they get an erection but it won't last or goes down. This is likely Veno-occlusive disorder or that hole in the tire. Blood flow comes in and an erection starts but then there is a "leak" in which certain tissue (the tunica or tire) has lost its integrity and is not as expansile or elastic. The valves that shut off escaping blood flow remain open so the blood goes back into the venous system and back to the heart leaving the penis soft. It has been shown that Testosterone may help the leak by improving the tissue structure of the tunica or tire- so less blood escapes or leaks. (See diagram)

Testosterone helps erectile dysfunction through:

- **Increased blood flow**
- **Better tissue structure to prevent leak**
- **Improved function of PDE5 inhibitors - sildenafil, tadalafil**

TAKE HOME POINT

Testosterone is helps erections on multiple fronts including blood flow and tissue elasticity

TESTOSTERONE DISSOCIATIVE PERCEPTION - MISSED EXPECTATIONS

Myth:

Testosterone replacement will always improve my energy

Reality:

Testosterone will improve energy, but many factors also play a significant role in feeling energetic

Many patients perceive energy and vitality as solely a testosterone function. The thought is that if we just raise the testosterone and energy should just go up. When patients come in for checkups and all of their numbers look good but they tell me "How come I still don't have that energy I used to have?" I explain to them, unfortunately, energy or the perception of energy is multifactorial. Many patients also have unrealistic expectations due to the internet or other sources which tout these. Testosterone is only one component of energy or feeling energetic. I have found that thyroid imbalances, stress, anemia, vitamin B-12 deficiency, overconsumption of caffeine or alcohol, sleep disturbances, all play a role. There is no one cure for decreased energy but I have found if the testosterone is low most patient's energy will improve once the testosterone levels are normalized. However in a minority of patients the energy does not return to their perceived satisfaction and that is what I have termed the "dissociative perception". Furthermore, societal impressions of heroes and athletes using anabolic steroids displaying superhuman strength feats and levels of energy also play into the idea of steroids being the panacea for low energy.

Reasons for lack of energy with normal testosterone/estrogen levels

- Stress (ok this is huge, cortisol fights testosterone)
- Thyroid conditions
- Sleep disturbances
- Anemia or low blood count
- Caffeine crash

─────────── TAKE HOME POINT ───────────

Testosterone only controls a part of energy and expectations must be clear prior to starting therapy

TESTOSTERONE AND PROSTATE ENLARGEMENT

Myth:

Testosterone causes a rise in PSA and you cannot take Testosterone if you have an enlarged prostate

Reality:

Testosterone does not cause a statistical rise in PSA and will not enlarge your prostate significantly long term

It was previously thought but now has been shown that testosterone does not increase Prostate Specific Antigen (PSA) levels. When patients are started on Testosterone therapy there is no or little change in PSA levels long term. In the short term, there may be a rise in PSA and mild enlargement of the prostate, but it is not associated with any increased risk of prostate cancer (more on that later).

It seems there is a saturation model in which despite the increases in blood testosterone levels, the prostate will be saturated and not take up anymore testosterone. This protects the prostate from higher testosterone blood levels. In fact, there is evidence to suggest that patients with low testosterone may have larger prostates due to inflammation and benign enlargement.

PSA levels should be ideally monitored every 6 months along with the other labs. If serum PSA were to rise significantly for 6 consecutive months or increase greater than 1.4 ng/mL in a year on T therapy, then consideration should be given for referral to a Urologist for a workup which may include other blood tests, specialized Magnetic Resonance Imaging (MRI) of the prostate or even prostate biopsy to exclude the possibility of occult prostate cancer.

TAKE HOME POINT

Prostate Specific Antigen levels should be monitored every 6 months in patients taking T therapy and any changes or significant increases investigated

---

Chapter 22

PROSTATE CANCER - A CONTROVERSIAL NEBULOUS CONUNDRUM IS NOW BECOMING CLEAR

Myth:

Testosterone causes prostate cancer, so if you have one, you better not risk it

Reality:

There is no evidence testosterone causes prostate cancer, furthermore evidence suggests, if in balance, it may prevent prostate cancer, and lastly it is safe in patients who have been successfully treated for prostate cancer

So you know how many times I have heard "Well my doctor said I shouldn't take testosterone because it causes prostate cancer. Does it?" The short answer is NO it does not cause prostate cancer. Some studies indicate estrogen may be the causative reason for the initial development for prostate cancer rather than testosterone. Nonetheless, if someone has an occult prostate cancer testosterone may subsequently cause it to grow. Prostate cancer is a change in the cells from organized to disorganized. Gene changes that allow cells to grow without being controlled or in check. Furthermore, our natural immune system tends to keep these rogue cells from proliferating. Certain environmental factors play more of a role with prostate cancer than does testosterone. Diet high in animal fats, exposure to pesticides, processed foods and yes, estrogen may be more important than testosterone in the development of prostate cancer.

Much of the concern about the risk of testosterone replacement or restorative therapy and prostate cancer is from the treatment we offer men with advanced or metastatic prostate cancer. The treatment for prostate cancer was established from research in the 1940's in which men whose testosterone production dropped, prostate cancer stopped growing. Furthermore, if testosterone was given it made the tumors grow. Since then, castration and medical castration has one of the mainstays of treatment for men with advanced and metastatic prostate cancer. These are forms of medical castration that significantly lower testosterone. But wait! It has been shown that men with low testosterone actually have a higher risk of aggressive prostate cancers.

So what is truly happening? It seems to be like everything in life - it is all about balance. Too low may be bad and of course too high may be bad. (See figure)

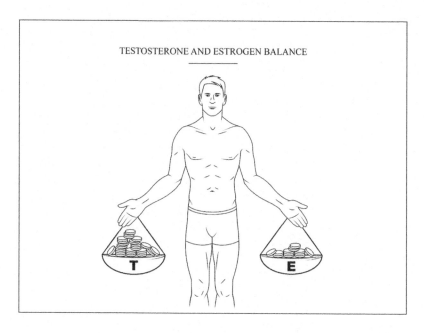

TESTOSTERONE AND ESTROGEN BALANCE

More and more studies are changing the way we think about testosterone replacement therapy after definitive treatment for prostate cancer. There seems to be no increased risk of prostate cancer recurrence in men treated with Testosterone replacement therapy vs those not treated.

Current recommendations are that patients with low risk prostate cancer, preoperative PSA of less than 10 ng/mL and Gleason score (the classification of aggressiveness of the cells, scale from 2-10) less than 8 and pathologic low stage of T1-T2 can be offered therapy after a year of curative treatment if PSA levels remain low.

There are currently no recommendations regarding Testosterone replacement therapy and patients undergoing active surveillance. Large quality of life benefits are again observed in these patients but too few limited studies support use in these men. I will say, however, that more experts are warming up to the idea of treatment in men undergoing active surveillance because of the indolence (slow growing pace) of the disease. Careful surveillance and caution of safety considerations must be kept in mind. The point of balance cannot be overstressed though.

──────────── TAKE HOME POINT ────────────

Testosterone in and of itself does not cause prostate cancer and can be used safely in certain men who have been treated for prostate cancer

LABORATORY VALUES - WHAT TO WATCH FOR AND WHAT YOUR DOCTOR SHOULD BE CHECKING

Myth:

Testosterone causes prostate cancer, so if you have one, you better not risk it

Reality:

Blood levels change, due to metabolism and medication clearance changes and labs should be checked frequently especially when initiating therapy then at least twice a year when stable dosing and levels are achieved

Your doctor should be obtaining and history, physical examination and checking certain labs at certain times. The history and physical should include historical questions of libido, erections, energy, urinary symptoms, anxiety or depression symptoms, and sleep patterns. Also one should inquire of blood disorders of increased clotting, stress, and prescription or any over-the-counter medications taken. Examination should include vital signs (especially blood pressure since this can be raised at times by testosterone therapy) testicular and breast exam and at least once yearly a digital rectal prostate examination.

I have seen some physicians start testosterone therapy and not check laboratory values for three or four months. Again as previously discussed, in my experience, four to six weeks of therapy is an ideal time to check blood work with any therapy instituted.

With clomiphene and HCG, I usually obtain labs in 4 weeks. With testosterone gels, I usually obtain labs at 3 to 4 weeks. With testosterone injections, I obtain labs at 4-6 weeks depending on the frequency of injections. I always tell patients to obtain labs in the middle of any injection interval. For instance if they take clomiphene citrate or HCG, on the "off" day. If they do injections then it would be at the midpoint of the two injections.

Labs to check upon initial evaluation

- FSH and LH
- Prolactin
- Estradiol
- Testosterone free and total
- CBC (complete blood count)
- PSA
- Serum Hormone binding globulin

Labs to check at least every 6 months

- Testosterone free and total
- Estradiol
- Hemoglobin and hematocrit -Red blood cell count
- Prostate Specific Antigen

––––––––––––– TAKE HOME POINT –––––––––––––

Checking labs more frequently in the beginning to dial in the numbers and desired effects is recommended along with 6 month lab draws once stable blood levels achieved

METABOLIC SYNDROME AND INSULIN METABOLISM MADE EASY - DON'T FALL INTO THE VORTEX

Myth:

Fat does not play role in Testosterone and Estrogen

Reality:

Fat plays a huge role, especially with Estrogen, which in turn affects how insulin works, which in turn affects how fat is made and so on…

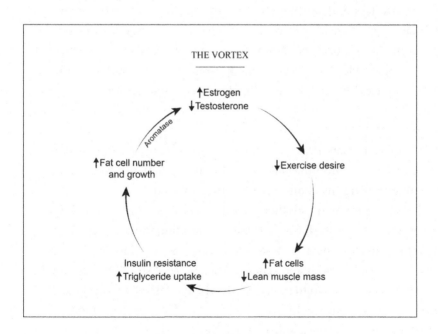

Metabolic syndrome is a term thrown around that even for medical professionals can be confusing. Think of it this way - if your fat around the midline - you have a high risk of having or developing metabolic syndrome and affecting the way insulin works, therefore increasing your risk for diabetes. Metabolic syndrome is a condition which includes obesity, increased triglycerides, insulin resistance and diabetes.

Yes, it is a vortex. Why do I call it this? Well, you see as we gain weight especially in our mid sections this creates an imbalance. It raises intra-abdominal fat (adipose tissue) that in turn converts more testosterone to estrogen. There is an enzyme in fat tissue called aromatase that is responsible for doing this. It has its highest concentrations in the intra-abdominal or belly fat. So think about it, your testosterone starts to go down naturally as we age then the intra-abdominal fat grows and expands, we lose lean muscle mass, our estrogen trends higher, more of our testosterone is bound by protein and then estrogen also at times in high concentrations completes with testosterone on the receptor level so our functional or free testosterone, the *gold*, goes lower and lower. Also, as testosterone goes down our level of energy suffers and we exercise less and fat tissue grows, increasing aromatase enzyme with subsequent insulin resistance, triglyceride storage suppression of T stimulating hormones from the brain and you guessed it, more fat cells! The cycle starts all over and becomes an increasingly vicious cycle - a vortex! Escaping the vortex is not easy but definitely can be done.

Let's face it there is a pandemic of men with larger "beer" bellies and extra intra-abdominal fat. But I see many patients who I joke with about losing my thanksgiving turkey in their belly but when I pinch their abdominal wall there is little fat between the skin and the underlying layer. It is all inside them surrounding their bowels. Well this is the worst kind of fat for testosterone, estrogen conversion, insulin resistance, triglyceride and cholesterol metabolism. Testosterone therapy has been shown to improve HB A1c and fasting blood glucose in as little as 3 months with potential further declines in 12 months. Patients with metabolic syndrome may see blood pressure and waist circumference benefits within 12 months.

Testosterone and Metabolic Syndrome

- Reduces fat
- Decreases triglycerides
- Improves insulin resistance
- Improves HB A1c
- Reduces estrogen conversion
- Reduces fat again

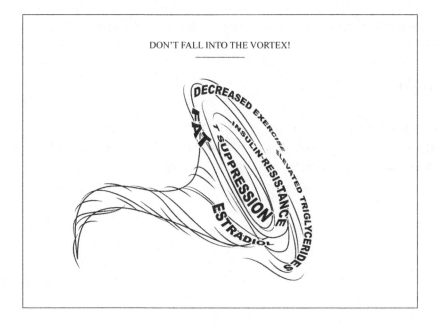

DON'T FALL INTO THE VORTEX!

DECREASED EXERCISE
ELEVATED TRIGLYCERIDES
FAT
INSULIN-RESISTANCE
SUPPRESSION
ESTRADIOL

——————— TAKE HOME POINT ———————

Metabolic syndrome is a self perpetuating phenomenon that may be helped with restorative or replacement T therapy

Chapter 25

ROLE OF TESTOSTERONE IN HEART DISEASE, CLOTTING AND LIPID PROFILE

Myth:

Testosterone causes heart attacks and strokes in otherwise healthy men.

Reality:

There is no solid or no compelling evidence that testosterone causes any increased risk of heart attack and stroke if used appropriately and may actually have beneficial heart effects in healthy men.

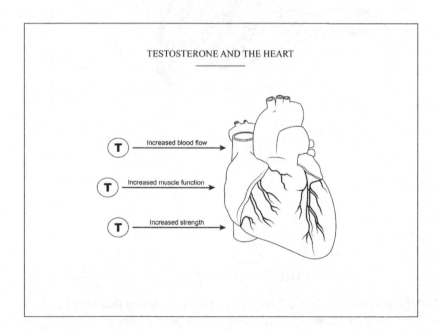

TESTOSTERONE AND THE HEART

T — Increased blood flow →

T — Increased muscle function →

T — Increased strength →

Since the US Food and Drug Administration (FDA) issued a warning of testosterone replacement products in 2015 there has been numerous studies showing the opposite is true: there are more beneficial effects than risks in terms of cardiac function and blood flow. Specifically the beneficial effects include improved heart failure, reduced inflammation and atherosclerosis and subsequent decreased risk of coronary artery disease. At the cellular level, there is purported improvements in atherosclerosis and vasodilation. Low Testosterone may also play a role in hardening of the arteries through mechanisms poorly understood but likely an influence on inflammation and vascular integrity, although these points are still controversial.

In older men, there is controversial evidence to suggest they are at risk for heart attack or stroke and these men should be evaluated medically for risk factors prior to beginning Testosterone replacement therapy. Long acting agents like the pellets may have decreased cardiovascular risk and may be an option for men who are at increased risk of cardiovascular events.

Bottom line - in most healthy men testosterone can be used safely with without significant increase in cardiovascular events however, in men with significant atherosclerotic disease or cerebrovascular disease caution should be taken and a discussion of risks and benefits of testosterone therapy must be discussed.

TESTOSTERONE AND CLOTTING

Myth:

Testosterone causes clotting in the deep veins

Reality:

There is potential risk of forming blood clots called deep vein thrombosis if there is a clotting disorder, so be aware and take precautions if there is history of clotting.

Men starting testosterone should be screened in a general history for clotting disorders including those of family members. Just as those used for evaluation for candidacy for oral contraceptives in females. However, again, the FDA has required that all testosterone products labels disclose potential risks of cardiovascular events like heart attack, stroke and clotting.

Bottom line - if you have any increased risk of clotting including a history of cancer talk to your doctor about testosterone therapy. If you choose to start testosterone therapy then at a minimum take a daily baby aspirin which may help prevent clotting or maybe testosterone therapy may be too risky for you.

TESTOSTERONE AND LIPID PROFILE

Myth:

Testosterone has no effect on cholesterol

Reality:

Testosterone lowers the bad cholesterol without changing the good

Multiple studies in the literature have shown the beneficial effects of testosterone on lipid profile. Testosterone replacement therapy in older men with low T has been shown to improve triglycerides, lower low density lipoprotien (LDL, the bad cholesterol) and raise or not change high density lipoprotein (HDL, the good cholesterol). It is still unclear whether these functions play any role in cardiovascular disease but one can imagine it would. I have also seen patients improve their lipid profiles, especially triglycerides and LDL.

Testosterone Cardiovascular benefits

- Protect heart from failure
- Improve blood flow to heart
- Improve lipid profile
- Reduce inflammation

Testosterone cardiovascular risks

- Any risk of coronary vascular disease or clotting check with your doctor!

--- TAKE HOME POINT ---

Testosterone may be beneficial to the heart and improve your cholesterol profile

Chapter 26

TESTOSTERONE AND THE BRAIN - COGNITION AND MOOD

Myth:

Testosterone does not affect the male brain

Reality:

Optimal levels of testosterone improves male brain cognitive function and mood

This area is where experience plays a role - both personal and professional. My personal experience with restoration was started because I knew something was not right. Furthermore, when I ran out of medication for a week or ten days I could feel a definite difference in mental clarity. Also, many men who I see as patients will describe a mental fog associated with low testosterone that only becomes more noticeable and pronounced if they run out or stop the replacement or restorative testosterone therapy.

Studies show there seems to be an optimal level in which Testosterone improves global cognitive function, specifically memory, attention and executive function. The optimal level will vary with everyone. Below that optimal level and above that level there are no gains in cognitive function or even negative effects on cognitive function may occur. (See inverted "U" diagram)

Some studies showing positive effects and protective effects in patients with cognitive impairment and leading to Alzheimers disease but this point is very controversial.

Overall, the level of improvement of cognitive function with men with low testosterone and restorative or replacement therapy may be subtle and controversial depending on the study. Reviews of the literature recognize that improvements or maintenance of cognitive abilities trend positive.

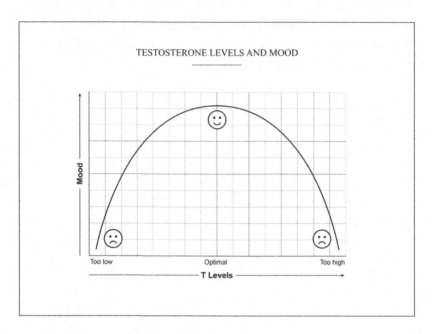

TESTOSTERONE LEVELS AND MOOD

TESTOSTERONE AND MOOD

Myth:

Testosterone levels do not affect mood

Reality:

Optimal testosterone levels can affect mood in certain patients

Testosterone has not been shown to improve major depressive disorder but can help in older men with age-induced depression.

This is another issue concerning balance. If testosterone levels are too low some men may have depressive disorders. If testosterone goes too high there is also depression and hypomania or steroid psychosis. So testosterone hormonal balance once again, the theme of this book, is important for healthy mood and outlook. I have seen many patients on anti-depression medications discontinue them once testosterone therapy was instituted. We are learning more about this but this scenario is quite commonplace now.

───────────────── TAKE HOME POINT ─────────────────

Testosterone seems to improve many facets of cognitive function and mood

Chapter 27

PRESCRIPTION MEDICATIONS - YES THEY CAN AFFECT YOU!

Myth:

Prescription medications do not affect hormones

Reality:

Many prescription medications affect hormones in the brain and testicles

Finasteride is a medication that is prescribed for enlarged prostate and in certain situations to reduce the risk of prostate cancer. It is a 5-alpha reductase enzyme inhibitor in target tissues including skin, hair and prostate. That is not the important thing to understand here though and we will get to the points in a minute. It is interesting to note that it was found to grow hair and then remarked as Propecia® for male pattern baldness in a lower dosage.

So this medication that causes hair growth, more importantly, changes your testosterone and estrogen profile and balance. Though a feedback loop it actually raises testosterone trapping by serum hormone binding globulin, raises estrogen levels, and decreases testosterone receptor activity causing potential reduction in libido, sperm production and ejaculatory volume. Although these side effects are usually temporary, I have seen patients who have experienced this long term side effect years after they have stopped the finasteride even though studies show return of hormonal and receptor balance. I have found men who are on Finasteride and testosterone replacement therapy are less likely to have this side effect.

A comprehensive list of medications that affect testosterone production and effectiveness is not possible since there are so many. The majority of antidepressants including Serotonin re-uptake inhibitors (SSRI) have effects on production and response of target tissue to testosterone. It is therefore important you share all medications, prescription or otherwise, you use with your doctor prior to starting any testosterone replacement or restorative therapy.

──────── TAKE HOME POINT ────────

Testosterone can be affected by multiple medications so it is important that a healthcare professional evaluate your medications prior to starting therapy

Chapter 28

OTHER MYTHS

MARIJUANA

Myth:

Marijuana lowers testosterone levels

Reality:

Marijuana has little effect on testosterone levels

I always thought marijuana had a negative effect on testosterone. As I researched further I found this was a controversial subject. Meaning some studies found a rise in testosterone and others lower or no change. There are receptors for THC (the active chemical in marijuana) in the male testicles that may play a role in testosterone production at least in the short term.

There is one study from from Denmark which shows it may raise testosterone levels and one from the US with no change in testosterone levels unless there was recent use which raised the level temporarily in younger men less than 30. **Bottom line** is that its effects testosterone still are controversial. Marijuana, surprisingly, has no effect on estrogen levels. Marijuana users do have decreased sperm counts and concentration in most studies.

ALCOHOL, OPIOIDS, AND TOBACCO

Myth:

Alcohol and drugs has no effect on hormone levels

Reality:

Alcohol opioids, and tobacco can lower testosterone levels and raise estrogen levels

Alcohol , opioids and tobacco (nicotine) affects hormone production in the brain that tells the testicles to make testosterone. Also, it directly affects the cells that make testosterone in the testicle. Long term alcohol use and opioid use also raises serum estrogen levels through increased aromatization. Many of these effects are reversible in short term use, that is, once the substance is discontinued in otherwise healthy men, testosterone returns to normal. Long term use, however, affects the brain to testicle pathways and irreversibly effects the testicles through atrophy and oxidative stress (think the opposite of antioxidants) So it is important for patients on T therapy to limit their alcohol intake.

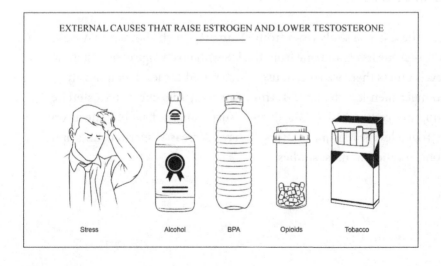

EXTERNAL CAUSES THAT RAISE ESTROGEN AND LOWER TESTOSTERONE

| Stress | Alcohol | BPA | Opioids | Tobacco |

WEIGHT LOSS

Myth:

Losing weight will raise my testosterone levels significantly

Reality:

Losing weight will bring down testosterone, but likely not to levels that will be desired and fulfilling.

Weight loss is a difficult process. Yes it can be done but here is the problem in men with low T. The desire and energy to exercise is usually nonexistent when a man has low T. So losing that weight can be extremely difficult - an uphill battle. Most men need to supplement their testosterone then also institute dietary changes and exercise regimens once they are feeling more themselves again with improved energy and the desire to workout. Most of these patients realize they have a problem but need a boost or help getting there. Weight loss helps with many aspects including insulin sensitivity and decreased fat leading to less aromatization and maximizing testosterone levels and efficiency.

SOY

Myth:

Soy is a phytoestrogen which lowers testosterone and raises estrogen

Reality:

Soy products do not lower testosterone levels nor raise estrogen levels

Admittedly before I started writing this I was one of those who thought soy at least raised estrogen levels. It is categorized as a phytoestrogen so it sounds intuitive. It was long thought that soy, as a phytoestrogen, lowered Testosterone and raised estrogen since animal studies indicated this phenomenon. It was thought that soy raised the serum hormone binding globulin which transports the testosterone molecule in the blood stream, hence lowering the free testosterone or the *gold*.

Human studies , however, have shown that there is no significant effects of soy protein on testosterone or free testosterone, because humans metabolize soy isoflavones (the active beneficial molecules) differently than animals. Soy has been shown to be protective against prostate cancer through preventive effects other than estrogen or testosterone changes. The bottom line is that soy has no effects on testosterone or estrogen.

BISPHENOL-A (BPA)

Myth:

All bottled water is safe because it is bottled.

Reality:

When BPA plastic is exposed to heat it is released into the contents of the bottle causing hormonal changes.

So we are told to drink more water. The issue is that our water sources in many parts of the US are not seen as pure and safe for drinking. So we turn to bottled water. The water is usually in plastic containers. Now water is not the only form of plastic container, but it is certainly one of the most common. Bisphenol-A (BPA) is a component of plastic containers and resin lining canned foods. Its use is ubiquitous in our society. When these plastic containers containing BPA are heated as in the sun or microwave for instance, the BPA leaches out into the food substance. BPA has been shown to lower testosterone and have estrogenic effects. Care must be taken that BPA-free does not include BPS which is a similar chemical compound and has equal estrogenic properties. Therefore, "BPA free" must be examined closely for phthalates and other BPA compounds in containers.

STRESS

Myth:

Stress does not affect our hormones - we can handle this

Reality:

Stress affects all of hormones to prepare our bodies for crisis

Stress plays a major role in all hormones. Cortisol is the most common stress hormone that is produced by the small adrenal glands just above the kidney. These steroids are responsible for regulating your response to different stressors like a lion chasing you in a "fight or flight". Cortisol tends to lower testosterone to block libido so the mind and body can deal with the crisis at hand. If cortisol is around it is usually the winner in this interplay. Cortisol will always trump testosterone.

Chronic stress can also lower testosterone through the same mechanism and feedback loops Although we would all like to reduce our daily stress, it seems to be ubiquitous in our society perhaps gleaning reasons of low Testosterone in younger males along with fertility issues. Reducing stress is one of the most beneficial ways to lower cortisol and raise functioning testosterone.

─────────────── TAKE HOME POINT ───────────────

Opioids, alcohol and stress lower testosterone levels while soy and marijuana do not affect testosterone levels

Chapter 29

GROWTH HORMONE, PEPTIDE THERAPY AND TESTOSTERONE

Myth:

Growth hormone will make me slimmer and leaner all by itself

Reality:

Growth hormone has limited abilities to reduce fat without Testosterone

L et me start by saying I prescribe very little growth hormone (GH) relative to testosterone. Not that I do not believe in it its just that I don't see patients who have clear identifiable indications for use. Growth hormone is indicated in frail men with muscle wasting, HIV positive men with muscle wasting and other growth hormone deficient men from causes like cancer and pituitary gland disorders. However, I thought it definitely deserves mention.

Growth Hormone is a master hormone which function is to prepare you for growth. Whether it be muscle growth, organ growth or bone growth. It mediates its effects through direct cell effects and a growth factor called Insulin-Like Growth Factor 1 (IGF-1). IGF-1 acts on muscle to increase cell volume and increase amino acid use. Furthermore, it makes fat cells break down stored fat to stimulate growth. IGF-1 also breaks down glycogen in the liver to glucose (fueling growth) and increases production of immune cells and neurotransmitters.

Most patients who are on GH are prescribed the medication by an anti-aging clinic or doctor. Admittedly very few patents who are on GH are not on some form of Testosterone at the time that I see them. There is evidence that Testosterone enhances GH effects on the body, especially fat reduction. There seems to be a synergism where one helps the other, more so than either alone.

Growth hormone alone has an average reduction of 12% fat mass and increase lean muscle mass along with increased exercise tolerance. If Testosterone is added, there can be an increase in fat mass reduction by up to 28%. The results of having Testosterone in combination of GH is similar to GH in higher doses, without the side effects. It is possible that lower doses of GH can be used when using Testosterone to achieve the same effects with out the collateral damage of high dose GH, including alterations in sugar metabolism, muscle and joint swelling, pain and irritability and carpal tunnel syndrome.

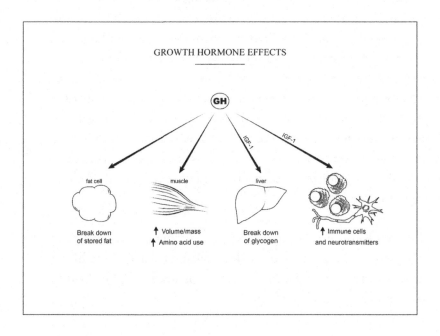

PEPTIDE THERAPY

Myth:

Peptide therapy is better than standard therapy and can be used safely in the US

Reality:

Currently in the United States Peptide therapy is for experimental use only and it has not been approved for use or administration in humans

Peptides are proteins manufactured to be injected that carry out desired effects on target tissue specifically and directly without being converted to other substances causing unwanted side effects. There has been increased interest in these manufactured proteins. They go directly to the tissue, bypass the middle man, and target the tissues desired. In contrast, hormones find the tissue and have that tissue make peptides or proteins that then carry out wanted effects. In the case of growth hormone, peptides (like IGF-1) are created at the target the tissue and then we see the clinical or metabolic effects. So the advantage of just injecting the actual protein that carries the effects on the tissue is clear. The other advantage is cost- these peptides can be created at a fraction of the cost of the actual recombinant hormones like growth hormone.

The results of limited studies on peptide therapy are intriguing with claims of less side effects due to less collateral metabolic pathways influenced as hormones do. More research is needed in this field to confirm or deny those claims.

Here is the kicker - in the United States peptide therapy is still considered experimental and labeled not for human use. Other countries do have this therapy approved and larger studies are needed to corroborate the touted results.

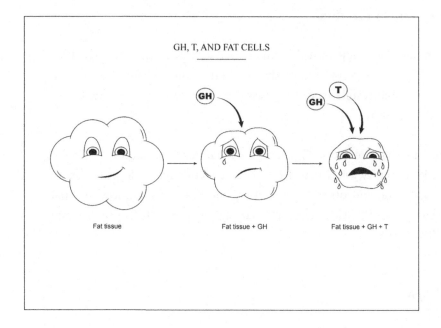

TAKE HOME POINT

Growth hormone has limited abilities to reduce fat without ideal testosterone levels

REFERENCES

Foreword by the editor

Johannes C, Araujo A, Feldman H, Derby C, Kleinman K, McKinlay J (200) Incidence of erectile dysfunction in men 40 to 69 years old: longitudinal results from the Massachusetts male aging study. J Urol 163(2): 460-3.

Feldman H, Longcope C, Derby C, Johannes C, Araujo A, Coviello A, Bremner W, McKinlay J (2002) Age trends in the level of serum testosterone and other hormones in middle-aged men: longitudinal results from the Massachusetts male aging study. J Clin Endrocrinol 87(2): 589-98.

Chapter 1

Feldman H, Longcope C, Derby C, Johannes C, Araujo A, Coviello A, Bremner W, McKinlay J (2002) Age trends in the level of serum testosterone and other hormones in middle-aged men: longitudinal results from the Massachusetts male aging study. J Clin Endrocrinol 87(2): 589-98.

Chapter 3

Balasubramanian, A, Thirumavalavan N, Srivatsav A, Yu J, Lipshultz L., Pastuszak A (2019)

Testosterone Imposters: An Analysis of popular online testosterone boosting supplements. J Sex Med16(2): 203-212.

Balasubramanian A, Thirumavalavan N, Srivatsav A, Yu J, Lipshultz L, Pastuszak A (2019)

An analysis of popular online erectile dysfunction supplements. J Sex Med 16(6): 843-852.

Almaiaman A, (2018) Effect of testosterone boosters on body functions: A case Report. Int J Health Sci 12(2) :86-90.

Enzyte Wikipedia Google search

Chalasani N, Fontana R, Bonkovsky H, Watkins P, Davern T, Serrano, J et al. (2008) Causes of clinical features, and outcomes from a prospective study of drug- induced liver injury in the United States. Gastroenterology 135: 1924-4.

Chapter 4

Kintz P, Cirimele V, Deveaux M, Ludes B (2000) Dehydroepiandrosterone (DHEA) and testosterone concentrations in human hair after chronic DHEA supplementation. Clinical Chemistry 46(3): 414.

Liu T, Lin C, Juang C, Ivy J, Kuo C (2013) Effect of acute DHEA administration on free testosterone in middle-aged and young men following high-intensity interval training. Eur J App Physiol 113(7): 1783-92.

Newman T (2018) How can DHEA benefit your health? Medical News Today, June.

Kritz-Silverstein D, von Muhlen D, Lughlin G, Bettencourt R (2008) Effects of Dehhydroepiandrosterone supplementation on cognitive function and quality of life: The DHEA and well-ness (DAWN) trial. J Am Geriatr Soc 56(7): 1292-1298.

Morales A, Hubrich R, Hwang J, Asakusa H, Yen S (1998) The effect of six months treatment with a 100 mg daily dose of dehydroepiandrosterone (DHEA) on circulating sex steroids, body composition and muscle strength in age-advanced men and women. 49(4): 421-32.

Von Muhlen D, Laughlinn G, Kritz-Silverman D, Barrett-Connor E (2007) The Dehydorepiandrosterone and well-ness (DAWN) study: research designs and methods. Contemp Clin Trials 28(2):153-68.

Villareal D (2002) Effects of dehydroepiandrosterone on bone mineral density: what implications for therapy? Treat Endocrinol 1(6): 349-57.

Brown G, Vukovich M, Sharp R, Reifenrath T (1999) Effect of oral DHEA on serum testosterone and adaptations to resistance training in young men. J Applied Physiol 87(6): 2274.

Sreekumaran Nair K, Rizza R, O'Brien P, Dhatariya K, Short K, Nehra A, Vittone J, Klee G, Basu A et al. (2006) DHEA in elderly women and DHEA or testosterone in elderly men. N Engl J Med 355:1647-1659.

Brown G, Vukovich M, King D (2006) Testosterone prohormone supplements. Med and Science in Sports and Exercise 38(8): 1451-1461.

King D, Sharp R, Vukovish M, Brown G, Reifenrath T, Nathaniel L, Parsons K (1999) Effect of oral androstenedione on serum testosterone and adaptations to resistant training in young men: a randomized controlled trial. JAMA 281(21): 2020-2028.

Leder B,Leblanc K, Longcope C, Lee H, Catlin D, Finkelstein J (2002) Effects of oral androstenedione administration on serum testosterone and estradiol levels in postmenopausal women. J Clin Endocrinol Metab 87(12): 5449-54.

Judge L, Bellar D, Hoover D, Biggs D, Leitzelar B, Craig B (2016) Effects of acute androstenedione supplementation levels in older men. Aging Male 19(3): 161-167.

Broeder C, Quindry J, Brittingham K, Panton L, Thomson J, Appakondu S, Bruel K, Byrd R, Douglas J, Earnest C, Mitchell C, Olson M, Roy T, Yarlagadda C (2000) The Andro project: physiological and hormonal influences of androstenedione supplementation in men 35 to 65 years old participating in a high-intensity resistance training program. Arch Int Med 160 (20): 3093-104.

Kovac J, Pan M, Arent A, Lipshultz L (2016) Dietary adjuncts for improving testosterone levels in hypogonadal males. American J of Men's Health 10(6): 109-117.

Brown G, Vukovich M, Martini E, Kohut M, Franke W, Jackson D, King D (2001) Effects of androstenedione-herbal supplementation on serum sex hormone concentrations in 30-to 59 year-old men. Int J Vitam Nutr Res 71(50): 293-301.

Prasad A, Mantzoros C, Beck F, Hess J, Brewer G (1996) Zinc status and serum testosterone of healthy adults. Nutrition 12(5): 344-8.

Hawkins V, Foster-Schubert K, Chubak J, Sorensen B, Ulrich C, Stancyzk F, Plymate S, Stanford J, White E, Potter J, McTiernan A (2008) Effect of exercise on serum sex hormones in men: A 12-month randomized clinical trial. Med Sci Sports Exerc 40(2): 223-233.

Yeo J, Cho S, Park S, Jo S, Ha J, Lee J Cho S, Park M (2018) Which exercise is better for increasing serum testosterone levels in patients with erectile dysfunction? World J Mens Health 36(2): 147-152.

Hayes L, Herbert P, Sculthorpe N, Grace F (2017) Exercise training improves free testosterone in lifelong sedentary aging men. Endocrin Connect 6(5): 306-310.

Wentz L, Berry-Caban C, Wu Q, Eldred J (2019) Vitamin D correlation with testosterone concentration in male US soldiers and veterans. J Military and Veterans' Health. 24(3): 1-13.

Lerchbaum E, Trummer C, Theiler-Schwetz V, Coleman M, Wolfler

M, Heijboer A, Pilz S, Obermayer-Pietsch B (2018) Effects of vitamin D supplementation on androgens in men with low testosterone levels: a randomized controlled trial. Eur J Nutr 10: 1007.

Pilz S, Frisch S, Koertke H, Kuhn J, Dreier J, Obermayer-Pietsch B, Wehr E, Zitterman A (2011) Effect of vitamin D supplementation on testosterone levels in men. Horm Metab Res 43(3): 223-5.

Lerchbaum E, Pilz S, Trummer C, Schwetz V, Parchernegg O, Heijboer A, Obermayer-Pietsch B (2017) Vitamin D and testosterone in healthy men: A randomized controlled trial. J Clin Endocrin Metab 102(11): 4292-4302.

Pilz S, Frisch S, Koertke H, Kuhn J, Dreier J, Obermayer-Pietsch B, Wehr E, Zitterman A (2011) Effect of vitamin D supplementation on testosterone levels in men. Hormone Metab Res 43(3): 223-5.

Lerchbaum E, Pilz S, Trummer C, Schwetz V, Pachernegg O, Heijboer A, Obermayer-Pietsch B (2017) Vitamin D and testosterone in healthy men: a randomized controlled trial. J Clin Endocrinol Metab 102(11): 4292-4302.

Chapter 5

Andersen M, Alvarenga, T, Mazaro-Costa R, Hachul H, Tufik S (2011) The association of testosterone, sleep, and sexual function in men and women. Brain Research 1416(6): 80-104.

Wittert G (2014) The relationship between sleep disorders and testosterone in men. Asian J Androl 16(2): 262-265.

Wittert G (2014) The relationship between sleep disorders and testosterone. Cur Opin Endocrinol Diabetes Obes 21(3): 239-43.

Patel P, Shiff B, Kohn T, Ramasamy (2019) Impaired sleep is associated with low testosterone in US adult males: results from the National Health and Nutrition Examination Survey. World J Urol 37(7): 1449-1453.

Andersen M, Tufik S (2008) The effects of testosterone on sleep and sleep-disordered breathing in men: its bidirectional interaction with erectile function. Sleep Med Rev 12(5): 365-79.

Barrett-Connor E, Dam T, Stone K, Harrison S, Redline S, Orwoll E (2008) The association of testosterone levels with overall sleep quality, sleep architecture, and sleep-disordered breathing. J Clin Endocrinol Metab 93(7): 2602-9.

Leproult R, Van Cauter E (2011) Effect of 1 week of sleep restriction on testosterone levels in young healthy men. JAMA 305(21): 2173-2174.

Chapter 6

Niedfeldt M (2018) Anabolic steroid effect on the liver. Curr Sports Med Rep 17(3): 97-102.

Perempongkosol S, Khupulsup K, Leelaphiwat S, Pavavattananusom S, Thingpradit S, Petchthong T (2016) Effects of 8-year treatment of long-acting testosterone undecanoate on metabolic parameters, urinary symptoms, bone mineral density, and sexual function in men with late-onset hypogonadism. J Sex Med 13(8): 1199-211.

Chapter 8

Aydogdu A, Swerdloff R (2016) Emerging medication for the treatment of male hypogonadism. Expert Opin Emerg Drugs 21(3): 255-66.

Hill S, Arutchelvam V, Quinton R (2009) Enclomiphene, an estrogen receptor antagonist for the treatment of testosterone deficiency in men. IDrugs 12(2): 109-19.

Wheeler K, Sharma D, Kavoussi P, Smith R, Costabile R (2019) Clomiphene citrate for the treatment of hypogonadism. 7(2): 272-276.

Taylor F, Levine L (2010) Clomiphene citrate and testosterone gel replacement therapy for male hypogonadism: efficacy and treatment cost. J Sex Med 7(1 Pt 1): 269-76.

Moskovic D, Katz D, Akhavan A, Park K, Mulhall J (2012) Clomiphene citrate is safe and effective for long-term management of hypogonadism. BJU Intl 110(10): 154-8.

Shabsigh A, Shabsign R, Gonzalez M, Liberson G, Fisch H, Goluboff E (2005) Clomiphene citrate effects on testosterone/estrogen ratio in male hypogonadism. J Sex Med 2(5): 716-21.

Dadhich P, Ramasamy R, Scovell J, Wilken N, Lipshultz L (2017) Testoserone versus clomiphene citrate in managing symptoms of hypogonadism in men. Indian J Urol 33(3): 236-240.

DiGorgio L, Sadeghi-Nejad H (2016) Off label therapies for testosterone replacement. Transl Androl Urol 5(6): 844-849.

Crosnoe-Shipley L, Elkelany O, Rahnema C, Kim E (2015) Treatment of hypogonadotropic male hypogonadism: Case-based scenarios. World J Nephrol 4(2): 245-253.

Habous M et al (2018) Clomiphene citrate and human chorionic gonadotropin are both effective in restoring testosterone in hypogonadism: a short-course randomized study. BJU Intl 122(5): 889-897.

Harman S et al (2015) Clomid in men with low testosterone with and without prior treatment. Clin trials.gov: 1-7.

Chapter 9

Hsieh T, Pastuszak A, Hwang K, Lipshultz L (2013) Concomitant intramuscular human chorionic gonadotropin preserves spermatogenesis in men undergoing testosterone replacement therapy. J Urol 189(2): 647-50.

Najari B Azoospermia with testosterone therapy despite concomitant intramuscular human chorionic gonadotropin. Rev Urol 20(3): 137-139.

Kim S, Ryu K, Hwang I, Jung S, Oh K, Park K (2011) Penile growth in response to human chorionic gonadotropin(HCG) treatment in patients with idiopathic hypogonadotropic hypogonadism. Chonnam Med 47(1): 39-42

Chapter 10

Lo E, Rodriguez K, Pastuszak A, Khera M (2018) Alternatives to testosterone therapy: A review. Sex Med Rev 6(1): 106-113.

Regitz-Zagrosek V, Wintermantel T, Schubert C (2007) Estrogens and SERMs in coronary heart disease. Curr Opin Pharmacol 7(2): 130-9.

Helo S, Wynia B, McCullough A (2017) "Cherchez La Femme": Modulation of estrogen receptor function with selective modulators: clinical implications in the field of urology. Sex Med Rev 5(3): 365-386.

Dias J, Shardell M, Carlson O, Melvin D, Caturegli G, Ferrucci L, Chia C, Egan J, Basaria S Testosterone vs. Aromatase inhibitor in older men with low testosterone: effects on cardio metabolic parameters.

Andrology 5(1): 31-40.

Tan R, Guay A, Hellstrom W (2014) Clinical use of aromatase inhibitors in adult males. Sex Med Rev 2(2):79-90.
Rambhatia A, Mills J, Rajfer J (2016) The role of estrogen modulators in male hypogonadism and infertility. Rev Urol 18(2): 66-72.

Chapter 11

Ullah M, Riche D, Koch C (2014) Transdermal testosterone replacement therapy in men. Drug Des Devel Ther 8: 101-112.

Chapter 12

Spratt D, Stewart I, Savage C, Craig W, Spack N, Chandler D, Spratt L, Eimicke T, Olshan, A (2017) Subcutaneous injection of testosterone is an effective and preferred alternative to intramuscular injection: Demonstration in female-to-male transgender patients. J Clin Endocrinol Metab 102(7): 2349-2355.

Borst S, Yarrow J (2015) Injection of testosterone may be safer and more effective than transdermal administration for combating loss of muscle and bone in older men. Am J Physiol Endorcrinol Metab 308(12): 1035-42.

Chapter 17

Soliman A, De Sanctis V, Yassin M (2017) Management of adolescent gynecomastia. Act Biomed 88(2): 204-213.

Chapter 19

Tharakan T, Miah S, Jayasena C, Minhas S (2019) Investigating the basis fo sexual dysfunction during late-onset hypogonadism. F1000res 8(1).

Rajfer J (2000) Relationship between testosterone and erectile dysfunction. Rev Urol 2(2):122-128.

Castela A, Vendeira P, Costa C (2011) Testosterone, endothelial health, and erectile function. ISRN Endocrinol 2011 839149.

Efesoy O, Cayan S, Akbay E (2018) The effect of testosterone replacement therapy on penile hemodynamics in hypogonadal men with erectile dysfunction, having veno-occlusive disease. Am J Mens Health 12(3): 634-638.

Elkoury F, Rambhatta A, Mills J, Rajfer J (2017) Cardiovascular health, erectile dysfunction, and testosterone replacement: controversies and correlations. Urology 110: 1-8.

Chapter 20

Tan R, Cook K, Reilly W (2015) High estrogen in men after injectable testosterone therapy: The low T experience. 9(3): 229-34.

Chapter 21

Kohn T, Mata D, Lipshultz L (2016) Effects of testosterone replacement therapy on lower urinary tract symptoms: a systematic review and meta-analysis. Eur Urol 69(6): 1083-1090.

Coward R, Simhan J, Carson C (2009) Prostate-specific antigen changes and in hypogonadal men treated with testosterone replacement therapy. BJU Intl 103(9): 1179-83.

Bell M, Campbell J, Joice G, Sopko N, Burnett A (2018) Shifting the paradigm of testosterone replacement therapy in prostate cancer. World J Mens Health 36(2): 103-109.

Debruyne F, Behre H, Roehborn C, Maggi M, Wu F, Shroder F, Jones T, Porst H, Hackett G, Wheaton O, Martin-Morales A, Muelman E, Cunningham G, Divan H, Rosen R (2017) Testosterone treatment is not associated with increased risk of prostate cancer or worsening lower urinary tract symptoms: prostate health outcomes in the registry of hypogonadal men.
BJU Intl 119(2): 216-224.

Xu X, Chen A, Hus H, Dalley A, Taylor B (2018) Current opinion on the role of testosterone in the development of prostate cancer: a dynamic model. BMC Cancer 26(15):806.

Harkonen P, Makela S (2004) Role of estrogens in development of prostate cancer. J Steroid Biochem Mol Biol 92(4): 297-305.

Bosland M (2005) The role of estrogens in prostate carcinogenesis: a rationale for chemoprevention. Rev Urol 7 (suppl 3): S4-S10.

Carruba G (2007) Estrogen and prostate cancer: an eclipse truth in an androgen-dominated scenario. J Cell Biochem 102(4): 899-911.

Nelles J, Wen-Yang H, Prins G. (2011) Estrogen action and prostate cancer. Expert Rev Endocrinol Metab 6(3): 437-451.

Pastuszak A, Khanna A, Badjwala N, Morgentaler A, Hult M, Conners W, Sarosdy M, Yang C, Carrion R, Lipshultz L, Khera M (2015)

Testosterone therapy after radiation therapy for low, intermediate and high risk prostate cancer. J Urol 194(5): 1271-6.

Kaplan A, Trinh Q, Sun M, Carter S, Nguyen P, Shih Y, Marks L, Hu J (2014) Testosterone replacement therapy following the diagnosis of prostate cancer: outcomes and utilization trends. J Sex Med 11(4): 1063-1070.

Kaplan A, Hu J, Morgentaler A, Mulhall J, Schulman C, Montorsi F (2016) Testosterne therapy in men with prostate cancer. Eur Urol 69(5): 894-903.

Golla V, Kaplan A (2017) Testosterone therapy on active surveillance and following definitive treatment for prostate cancer. Curr Urol Rep 18(7): 49.

Sarosdy M (2007) Testosterone replacement therapy for hypogonadism after treatment of early prostate cancer with brachytherapy. Cancer 109(3): 536-41.

Kim M, Kim J, Kim J, Lee S, Song C, Jeong I, Hong J, Kim C, Ahn H (2018) Association between serum levels of insulin-like growth factor-1, bioavailable testosterone, and pathologic Gleason score. Cancer Med 7(8): 4170-4180.

Chapter 25

Baillargeon J, Urban R, Morgentaler A, Glueck C, Baillargeon G, Sharma G, Kuo Y (2015) Risk of venous thromboembolismin in men receiving testosterone therapy. Mayo Clinic Proceedings 90(8): 1038-1045.

Glueck C, Wang P (2014) Testosterone therapy , thrombosis, thrombophilia, cardiovascular events. Metabolism 63(8): 989-984.

Sharma R, Oni O, Chen G, Sharma M, Dawn B, Sharma R, Parashara D, Savin V, Barua R, Gupta K (2016) Association between testosterone replacement therapy and the incidence of DVT and pulmonary embolism: a retrospective cohort study of the veterans administration database. Chest 150(3): 563-571.

Moll S (2017) Testosterone therapy: risk factor for venous thromboembolism. Hematologist 14(2): 1.

Houghton D, Alsawas M, Barrionuevo P, Tello M , Farah W, Beuschel B, Prokop L, Layton J, Murad M, Moll S (2018) Testosterone therapy and venous thromboembolism: a systematic review and meta-analysis. Throm Res 172: 94-103.

Maritnez C, Suissa S, Rietbrock S, et al. (2016) Testosterone treatment and risk of venous thromboembolism: population based case-control study. BMJ: 355. Comments by Strum S

Glueck C, Goldenberg N, Wang P (2018) Testosterone therapy, thrombophilia, venous thromboembolism, and thrombotic events. J Clin Med 8(1) E11.

Herring M, Oskui P, Hale S, Kloner R (2013) Testosterone and the cardiovascular system: a comprehensive review of the basic science literature. J Am Heart Association 2(4) e000272.

Chrysant S, Chrysant G (1995) Cardiovascular benefits and risks of testosterone replacement therapy in older men with low testosterone. Hosp Pract 46(2):47-55.

Traish A, Saad F, Feeley R, Guay A (2009) The dark side of testosterone deficiency: III. Cardiovascular disease. J Androl 30(5): 477-94.

Tanna M, Schwartzbard, Berger J, Underberg J, Gianos E, Weintraub H (2018) Management of hypogonadism in cardiovascular patients: What are the implications of testosterone therapy on cardiovascular morbidity? Urol Clin N Am 43(2): 247-60.

Anawalt B, Yeap B (2018) Conclusions about testosterone therapy and cardiovascular risk. Asian J Androl 20(2): 152-153.

Elagizi A, Kohler T, Lavine C (2018) Testosterone and cardiovascular health. Mayo Clin Proc 93(1): 83-100.

Traish A (2016) Testosterone therapy in men with testosterone deficiency: Are the benefits and cardiovascular risks real or imagined? Am J Phys Regul Integr Comp Physiol 311(3): 566-73.

Hwang K, Miner M (2015) Controversies in testosterone replacement therapy: testosterone and cardiovascular disease. Asian J Androl 17(2): 187-91.

Monroe A, Does A. (2013) The effect of androgen on lipids. Curr Opin Endocrinol Diabetes Obes 20(2): 132-9.

Wickrammatilake C, Mohideen M, Pathirana C (2013) Association of serum testosterone with lipid abnormalities patients with angiographically proven coronary artery disease. Indian J Endocrinol Metab 17(6): 1061-1065.

Nathan L, Shu W, Dinh H, Mukherjee T, Wang X, Lusis A, Chaudhurt G. (2001) Testosterone inhibits early atherogenesis by conversion to estradiol: critical role of aromatase. Proc Natl Acad Sci 98(6): 3589-93.

Vermeulen A, Kaufman J, Geomaere S, van Pottelberg I. (2002) Estradiol in elderly men. Aging Male 5(2): 98-102.

Vodo S, Bechi N, Petroni A, Muscoli C, Aloisi AM (2013) Testosterone-induced effects on lipids and inflammation. Mediators Inflamm 31.

Zgliczynski S, Ossowski M, Slowinska-Srzednicka j, Brzezinska A, Zgliczynski W, Soszynski P, Chotkowska E, Srzednicki M Sadowski

Z. (1996) Effect of testosterone replacement therapy on lipid and lipoproteins in hypogonadal and elderly men. Atherosclerosis 121(1): 35-43.

Miner M, Morgentaler A, Khera M, Traish A (2018) The state testosterone therapy since the FDA's 2015 labeling changes: indications and cardiovascular risk. Clin Endocrinol 89(1): 3-10.

Sigalos J, Pastuszak A, Khera M (2018) Hypogonadism: Therapeutic risks, benefits, and outcomes. Med Clin N America 102(2) : 361-372.

Chapter 26

Atwi S, McMahon D, Scharfman H, MacLusky, N. (2016) Androgen Modulation of Hippocampal Structure and Function. Neuroscientist 22 (1): 46-60.

Beauchet, O (2006) Testosterone and cognitive function: Current clinical evidence of a relationship. Eur J Endocrinol, 155 (6): 773-81.

Hua J, Hildreth K, Pelak V. (2016) Effects of Testosterone Therapy on Cognitive Function in Aging: A Systematic Review. Cogn Behav Neurol 29(3): 122-138.

Gruenewald D, Matsumoto A (2003) Testosterone supplementation therapy for older men: potential benefits and risks. J Am Geriatr Soc 51(1): 101-115.

Amanatkar H, Chibnall J, Seo B, Manepalli J, Grossberg G (2014) Impact of exogenous testosterone on mood: a systematic review and meta- analysis of randomized placebo -controlled trials. Ann Clin Psychiatry 26(1): 19-22.

Johnson J, Nachtigall L, Stern T. (2013) The effect of testosterone levels on mood in men: a review. Psychosomatics 54(6): 509-514.

Spitzer M, Basaria S, Travison T, Davda M, DeRogatis L, Bhasin S (2013) The effect of testosterone on mood and well-being men with erectile dysfunction in a randomized, placebo-controlled trial. Andrology 1(3): 475-482.

Resnick M, Matsumoto A, Stephens-Shields A, Ellenberg S, Gill T, Shumaker S, Pleasants D, Barrett-Conner E et al. (2017) Testosterone treatment and cognitive functioning older men with low testosterone and age-associated memory impairment. 21:317(7): 717-727.

Celec P, Ostatnikova D, Hodosy J (2015) On the effects of testosterone and brain behavioral functions. Front Neurosci 9: 12.

Seidman S, Weiser M (2013) Testosterone and mood in aging men. Psychiatr Clin N Am 36: 177-182.

Chapter 27

Traish A, Krakowsky Y, Doros G, Morgentaler A (2019) Do 5-Alpha reductase inhibitors raise circulating serum testosterone levels? A comprehensive review and meta-analysis to explaining paradoxical results. Sex Med Rev 7(1) 95-114.

Yuval R, Czarnowicki T, Ziotogorski A (2009) Finasteride induced gynecomastia: case report nd review of the literature, Int J Trichology 1 (1): 27-29.

Roerborhn C, Lee M, Meehan A, Waldstrelcher J (2003) Effects of finasteride on serum testosterone and body mass index in men with benign prostatic hyperplasia. Urology 62(5): 894-899.

Mysore V (2012) Finasteride and sexual side effects. Indian Dermatol Online J 3(1): 62-65.

Traish A (2017) Negative impact of testosterone deficiency and 5alpha-reductase inhibitor therapy on metabolic and sexual function in men. Adv Exp Med Biol 1043:473-526.

Chapter 28

Fior, K (2009) Bisphenol A mimics estrogen, phthalates target testosterone. Med Page Today pg 1-3.

Rettner, R. (2013) BPA linked with lower Testosterone. Live Science May 8: pg 1-5.

Galloway T, Cipelli R, Guralnick, J, Ferrucci L, Bandinelli S, Corsi A, Money C, McCormack P, Melzer D (2010) Daily Bisphenol A excretion and associations with sex hormone concentrations: Results from the InChIANTI adult population study. Env Health Perspectives 10: 1289.

Scinicariello F, Buser M. (2016) Serum testosterone concentrations and urinary Bisphenol A, Benzophenone-3, Triclosan, Paraben levels in male and female children and adolescents: NHANES 2011-2012. Env Health Perspectives 124(2): 1898-1904.

Nakamura D, Yanagiba Y Duan Z, Ito Y, Okamura A, Asaeda N, Tagawa Y, Li C, Zhang S, Naito H Ramdhan, D Kamijima, M Nakajima T (2010) Bisphemol A may cause testosterone reduction by adversely affecting both testis and pituitary systems similar to estradiol. Toxicol Lett 15;194 1-2: 16-25.

Minguez-Alarcon, L Hauser, R Gaskins, A. (2016) Fertil Steril 106(4): 864-870.

Cody H, Mobley B, Vann C, Romero M, Roberson M, Mumford P, Kephart W, Healy J, Patel R, Osburn S et al. (2018) Soy protein supplementation is not androgenic or estrogenic in college-aged men when combined with resistance exercise training. Sci Rep 8: 1038.

Hamilton-Reeves J, Vazquez G, Duval S, Phipps W, Kurzer M, Messina M (2010) Clinical studies show no effects of soy protein or isoflavones on reproductive hormones in men: results of a meta-analysis. Fertil Steril 94(3): 997-1007.

Messina M (2016) Soy and health update: evaluation of the clinical and epidemiologic literature.
Nutrients 8(12): 754.

Messina M, Hamilton-Reeves J, Kurzer M, Phipps W (2007) Effects of soy protein on testosterone levels. Cancer Epidemiol Biomarkers and Prevention. 16(12): 1158.

Jargin S (2014) Soy and phytoestrogens: possible side effects. Gen Med Sci 12(18) Doc 18.

Messina M (2010) Soybean isoflavone exposure does not have feminizing effects on men: a critical examination of the clinical evidence. Fertil Steril 93(7): 2095-104.

Fore K (2009) Bisphenol A mimics estrogen, phthalates target testosterone. Medpage Today.

Rettner R, BPA linked with lower testosterone. livescience.com

Scinicarelllo F, Buser M (2015) Serum testosterone concentrations and urinary Bisphenol A, Benzophenone-3, Triclosan, and Paraben levels male and female children and adolescents: NHANES 2011-2012. Environ Health Perspect 124(12): 1898-1904.

MInguez-Alarcon L, Hauser R, Gaskins A (2016) Effects of Bisphenol A on male and couple reproductive health: a review. Fertil Steril 106(4): 864-870.

Thistle J, Graubard B, Braunlin M, Vesper H, Trabert B, Cook M, McGlynn K (2017) Marijuana use and serum testosterone concentrations among U.S. males. Andrology 5: 732-738.

Herclerode J (1984) Endocrine effects of marijuana in the male: preclinical studies. NIDA Res Monogr 44: 46-64.

Vidot D, Prado G, Hlaing V, Florez H, Arheart K, Messiah S (2016) Metabolic syndrome among marijuana users in the United States: An analysis of national health and nutrition examination survey data. Am J Med 129(2): 173-9.

Duca Y, Aversa A, Condorelli R, Calogero A, La Vignera S (2019) Substance abuse and male hypogonadism. J Clin Med 8(5): 732.

Block R, Farinpour R, Schlechte J (1991) Effects fo chronic marijuana use on testosterone, luteinizing hormone, follicle stimulating hormone, prolactin and cortisol in men and women. Drug Alcohol Depend 28(2): 121-8.

Gundersen T, Jorgensen N, Andersson A, Bang A, Nordkap L, Skakkebaek N, Priskorn L, Juul A, Jensen T (2015) Association between use of marijuana and male reproductive hormones and semen quality: A study among 1,215 healthy young men. Am J Epidemiol 182(6): 473-481.

Emanuele M, Emanuele N (2001) Alcohol and the male reproductive system. Alcohol Res Health 25(4): 282-7.

Chapter 29

Ginzburg E, Lin A, Sigler M, Olsen D, Klimas N, Mintz A (2008) Testosterone and growth hormone normalization: a retrospective study of health outcomes. J Multidiscip Healthcare 1: 79-86.

Ginzburg E, Klimas N, Parvus C, Life J, Willix R, Barber M, Lin A, Comite F. (2010) Long-term safety of testosterone and growth hormone supplementation: a retrospective study of metabolic, cardiovascular, and oncologic outcomes. J Clin Med Res 2(4): 159-166.

Gibney J, Welters T, Maises M, Smythe G, Umpleby A, Ho K. (2003) Testosterone enhances the effect of growth hormone (GH) to increase IGF-1 but exerts an anabolic effect that is independent of GH action. Endocrine Abstracts

Birzniece V, Meinhardt U, Umpleby M, Handelsman D, Ho K. (2004) Interaction between testosterone and growth hormone in whole-body protein anabolism occurs in the liver. Endocrine Research.

Maran M, Sivakumar R, Ravisankar B, Valli G, Ravichandran K, Arunakaran J, Aruldhas M (2000) Growth hormone directly stimulates testosterone and oestradiol secretion by rat leydig cells in vitro and modulates effects of LH and T3. Endocr J 47(2): 111-118.

Giannoulis M, Sonksen P, Umpleby M, Breen L, Pentecost C, Whyte M, McMillan V, Bradley C, Martin F (2006) The effects of growth hormone and/or testosterone in healthy elderly men: and randomized controlled trial. J Clin Endocrinol and Metabolism 91(2): 477-484.

Chen R (2016) Human growth hormone and sex steroid supplementation. Library podcast blog. July 28 2016.

INDEX

Made in United States
North Haven, CT
18 July 2023

39226029R00082